Progress in Pain Research and Management
Volume 25

Opioids and Pain Relief:
A Historical Perspective

Mission Statement of IASP Press®

The International Association for the Study of Pain (IASP) is a nonprofit, interdisciplinary organization devoted to understanding the mechanisms of pain and improving the care of patients with pain through research, education, and communication. The organization includes scientists and health care professionals dedicated to these goals. The IASP sponsors scientific meetings and publishes newsletters, technical bulletins, the journal *Pain*, and books.

The goal of IASP Press is to provide the IASP membership with timely, high-quality, attractive, low-cost publications relevant to the problem of pain. These publications are also intended to appeal to a wider audience of scientists and clinicians interested in the problem of pain.

Progress in Pain Research and Management
Volume 25

Opioids and Pain Relief: A Historical Perspective

Editor

Marcia L. Meldrum, PhD

John C. Liebeskind History of Pain Collection,
Louise M. Darling Biomedical Library, and
Department of History, University of California, Los Angeles,
Los Angeles, California, USA

IASP PRESS® • SEATTLE

Timely topics in pain research and treatment have been selected for publication, but the information provided and opinions expressed have not involved any verification of the findings, conclusions, and opinions by IASP®. Thus, opinions expressed in *Opioids and Pain Relief: A Historical Perspective* do not necessarily reflect those of IASP or of the Officers and Councillors.

No responsibility is assumed by IASP for any injury and/or damage to persons or property as a matter of product liability, negligence, or from any use of any methods, products, instruction, or ideas contained in the material herein. Because of the rapid advances in the medical sciences, the publisher recommends that there should be independent verification of diagnoses and drug dosages.

Library of Congress Cataloging-in-Publication Data

Opioids and pain relief : a historical perspective / editor, Marcia L. Meldrum.
    p. ; cm. -- (Progress in pain research and management ; v. 25)
  Includes bibliographical references and index.
  ISBN 0-931092-47-7 (alk. paper)
    1. Analgesics--History. 2. Opioids--History. 3. Narcotics--History. I. Meldrum, Marcia. II. Series.
  [DNLM: 1. Narcotics--history. 2. Analgesics, Opioid--history. 3. Ethics, Medical. 4. Pain--drug therapy. 5. Pain--history. QV 11.1 O61 2003]
  RM319.O657 2003
  615'.783'09--dc21

                                           2003051121

Published by:

IASP Press
International Association for the Study of Pain
909 NE 43rd Street, Suite 306
Seattle, WA 98105-6020 USA
Fax: 206-547-1703
www.iasp-pain.org
www.painbooks.org

Printed in the United States of America

Contents

Contributing Authors

Caroline J. Acker, PhD *Department of History, Carnegie Mellon University, Pittsburgh, Pennsylvania, USA*

Huda Akil, PhD *Departments of Neuroscience and Psychiatry and Mental Health Research Institute, University of Michigan, Ann Arbor, Michigan, USA*

David Clark, PhD *Trent Palliative Care Centre, University of Sheffield, Sheffield, United Kingdom; currently Institute for Health Research, Lancaster University, Lancaster, United Kingdom.*

Michael J. Cousins, MD, FFPMANZCA, FANZCA, FRCA *Department of Anaesthesia and Pain Management, Royal North Shore Hospital; Pain Management Research Institute, Royal North Shore Hospital and University of Sydney, Sydney, New South Wales, Australia*

Nessa Coyle, PhD, NP, FAAN *Department of Neurology, Pain and Palliative Care Service, Memorial-Sloan-Kettering Cancer Center, New York, New York, USA*

June L. Dahl, PhD *Department of Pharmacology, University of Wisconsin Medical School, Madison, Wisconsin, USA*

Christina Faull, FRCP, MD *Department of Palliative Care, University Hospital, Birmingham, United Kingdom; currently Department of Palliative Care, Leicester Royal Infirmary, Leicester, United Kingdom*

Martha Stoddard Holmes, PhD *Department of Literature and Writing Studies, California State University, San Marcos, California, USA*

John D. Loeser, MD *Departments of Neurological Surgery and Anesthesiology, University of Washington, Seattle, Washington, USA*

Marcia L. Meldrum, PhD *John C. Liebeskind History of Pain Collection, Louise M. Darling Biomedical Library, and Department of History, University of California, Los Angeles, Los Angeles, California, USA*

Alexander Barnes Nicholson, MBBS *Department of Palliative Care, University Hospital, Birmingham, United Kingdom; currently Compton Hospice, Wolverhampton, United Kingdom*

Kenner C. Rice, PhD *Laboratory of Medicinal Chemistry, National Institute of Diabetes and Digestive and Kidney Diseases, National Institutes of Health, Department of Health and Human Services, Bethesda, Maryland, USA*

Walton O. Schalick III, MD, PhD *Departments of Pediatrics and History, Washington University in St. Louis, St. Louis, Missouri, USA*

Mark Swerdlow, DM *Deceased; formerly Regional Northwest Pain Centre, University of Manchester, Manchester, United Kingdom*

Preface

Opioids have been the mainstay of pain relief for centuries, yet the 21st-century pain field continues to debate their appropriate use in chronic and severe acute pain. The symposium that gave birth to this book, with the theme "Opioids, the Janus Drugs, and the Relief of Pain," was sponsored by the John C. Liebeskind History of Pain Collection and took place at the University of California Los Angeles on August 23–24, 2002. Many people questioned the phrase "Janus Drugs": What was the allusion? We were trying to describe the dual nature of opioids by using the image of the Roman god Janus who faced in two directions: on the one hand, these powerful analgesics ease the suffering of chronic and severe pain; on the other, their overuse or abuse can lead to the degradation of body and mind. What other drug has such a rich history and is so interwoven with the imagery of the best and worst in humanity? Janus was the god of doors and gates, also a fitting image as it suggests the importance of the spinal gate in pain history, the relationship between the opioid drugs and their receptor gates, and the door we were trying to open into a new historical topic. Several excellent historical works have presented the history of opiates as addictive substances, but I know of none that focuses specifically on the history of opioids in pain relief. Hence our symposium and this book.

As with the first Liebeskind Collection History of Pain Symposium in 1998, "Pain and Suffering in History," in organizing this symposium we were determined to bring together scientists and historians working in many different fields with complementary perspectives to share and debate. Among these eminent scholars were Walton Schalick, a pediatrician who is also an expert in French medieval medicine; Martha Stoddard Holmes, who reads 19th-century medical works for their literary interest; Caroline Acker, the leading American historian of addiction science in the early 20th century; Kenner Rice, NIDDK chemist and developer of the NIH opiate total synthesis; David Clark, whose Hospice History Project at the University of Sheffield has been documenting the fascinating origins of the modern hospice; Huda Akil, whose observations on stimulation-produced analgesia provided one of the keys to unlocking the secrets of the endogenous opioids; Christina Faull and Alexander Nicholson, two British specialists in palliative medicine who have researched the history of their field; Michael Cousins, our colleague from Australia who was a pioneer in the spinal administration of opioids; the late Mark Swerdlow, consultant to the World Health Organization on the groundbreaking Cancer Pain Relief Program; June Dahl, inspiration and motive force behind the American Alliance of Cancer Pain Initiatives; and Nessa Coyle, whose research is based on her wealth of nursing experience on the Pain and Palliative Care Service at Memorial-Sloan-Kettering.

John Loeser opened the symposium with inimitable flair and insight, and I have offered a closing chapter that draws on much of what I learned during those exciting two days. Our audience responded to the interdisciplinary format with enthusiastic and provocative comments and questions. All the chapters presented in this volume have benefited from the collegial interaction at the symposium, as well as from the suggestions of outside readers in the case of the historical chapters, and we are very grateful to all.

I owe a special debt of thanks to the Liebeskind Collection and UCLA Biomedical Library Staff, who met all my demands and requests with efficiency, grace, and good will during the two years we planned the symposium: Katharine Donahue, my co-director; Russell Johnson, our archivist, right hand, and left hand; and Teresa Johnson, Elaine Takahashi, Nadene McDonald, and Michelle Kasik. In making this book happen, Elizabeth Endres has been an intelligent and patient editor, and Roberta Scholz an invaluable support. We are grateful to Purdue Pharma, Ltd., for the unrestricted educational grant that made the symposium possible.

We remember John Liebeskind in everything we do and we dedicate this book to his memory.

MARCIA L. MELDRUM

IASP Press acknowledges the generous support of Endo Pharmaceuticals for the publication of this book.

Opioids and Pain Relief: A Historical Perspective,
Progress in Pain Research and Management, Vol.
25, edited by Marcia L. Meldrum, IASP Press,
Seattle, © 2003.

1

Opiophobia and Opiophilia

John D. Loeser

Departments of Neurological Surgery and Anesthesiology,
University of Washington, Seattle, Washington, USA

This volume is a collective effort to address the historical and contemporary use of opium and its derivatives as treatment for the relief of pain. It is not an attempt to provide prescribing information; rather, the editor has called upon historians, philosophers, and care providers to discuss issues relating to the administration of opiates by those given the awesome responsibility of treating pain and suffering. Although opiates have been used for medicinal purposes for at least 3,000 years, we still do not adequately understand their effects upon biology or psychology. Nor is there agreement in our cultures on the proper role of these drugs for medicinal or nonmedicinal usage (Davenport-Hines 2002). Voltaire summarized our predicament when he wrote: "Doctors pour drugs, of which they know little, for diseases, of which they know less, into patients—of which they know nothing."

In the 40 years that I have been treating patients with chronic pain, nothing has changed more than the use of opiates. In the 1960s and 1970s, it was considered inappropriate for any patient suffering from chronic pain to receive long-term treatment with any opiate drug, regardless of dose. The early pain clinics were inundated with patients who were receiving multiple opiates from multiple physicians and yet still complained bitterly of pain (Turner et al. 1982). Physicians spent considerable time trying to help patients to stop using these drugs and to engage in a more active road to restoration of function. In this era, nurses attempted to give postoperative patients the minimum amount of opiates that they deemed appropriate to the patient's needs. Oral and intramuscular routes of administration were common, intravenous administration was rare, and intrathecal routes not yet considered.

Improvements in the management of cancer pain with opiates, promoted by a small group of specialists in the 1980s, have been extrapolated to all chronic pain patients (Foley 1985). Now we have no upper dosing limit, and many patients with chronic pain are receiving long-term opiate administration. Patient-controlled analgesia is widely used for postoperative pain; the intrathecal route is common for both acute and chronic pain; and long-term treatment with morphine and other opiates has, in some quarters, replaced pain management and functional restoration. Data to support these dramatic changes in the prescription of opiates are scarce, at best.

The origin of the use of opiates has been lost in antiquity. The Ebers Papyrus of 1552 B.C.E. includes the earliest known written reference to opiates, which has been translated as, "The goddess Isis gave the juice of the poppy to Ra, the sun god, to treat his headache." Writings from seventh-century B.C.E. Sumeria refer to poppy juice. Opiates were used medicinally and probably recreationally in the Greek and Roman eras; as Schalick indicates in this volume, they were known and used during the medieval period in Europe. Their cultivation probably began in Asia Minor and spread to India and China along traditional trade routes.

By the 19th century, European traders, sailing to China to buy tea, silk, and porcelain, wished to bring goods to sell there, rather than make the long voyage with empty cargo holds. The English and the Portuguese developed a market for opium in the Chinese coastal ports. By 1840 the Emperor had become alarmed and wrote a letter to Queen Victoria, asking her to halt this trade, which he said was poisoning his people. The English responded by waging two wars with China to force the government to allow the unfettered importation and sale of opium. Meanwhile, the use of opiates in Europe and America was rapidly increasing. Opiates and cocaine could be found in many patent medicines, herbals, and tonics. At this time, the term "pipe dream" was introduced into English.

> O just, subtle, and all-conquering opium! That, to the hearts of rich and poor alike, for the wounds that will never heal, and for the pangs of grief that 'tempt the spirit to rebel' bringest an assuaging balm; and through one night's heavenly sleep callest back to the guilty man the visions of his infancy, and hands washed from pure blood. Thou only givest these gifts to man; and thou hast the keys of Paradise." (De Quincey 1971)

Opium was cheap and readily available in the Western world at the beginning of the 20th century; its widespread use produced much less misery than did alcohol. "Opium ... the Creator himself seems to prescribe, for we often see the scarlet poppy in the cornfields, as if it were foreseen that wherever there is hunger to be fed there must also be pain to be soothed" (Holmes 1961). We should not forget that tobacco, caffeine, alcohol, and marijuana, like opium and its derivatives, are all psychoactive drugs whose rules for use are not based upon medical facts; instead they are governed by sometimes capricious social conventions. "That humanity at large will ever be able to dispense with Artificial Paradises seems very unlikely" (Huxley 1963).

The 1914 Harrison Narcotic Act in the United States, and similar laws of that era in other countries, restricted the legal use of opiate drugs to medication prescribed by a physician. Since then, physician pronouncements about opiates usually reflect social conventions and are rarely based upon scientific evidence. National and state governments have enacted drug use laws that have criminalized behaviors that were once private business (Eldridge 1962; King 1972). Physicians are always prisoners of their referral patterns. Through personal experience alone, a physician cannot know the incidence or prevalence of a disease or the responses to treatment of the population at large.

Physicians in the modern era use potent opiates almost exclusively to treat pain. Research has provided no evidence that a significant proportion of pain patients abuse opiates given for pain relief. Physicians should not base their usage of opiates in pain management upon propaganda, yet they must not be oblivious to the potential for illegal use and diversion. Some have questioned why, in the United States, ownership of a lethal weapon such as a gun is protected and the owner not liable if it is used in a homicide, whereas possession of an opiate drug can lead to jail time.

Nor is there evidence that opiates are the best available treatment for all who suffer with chronic pain. Not all pains are the same, and it is necessary to discriminate between acute and chronic pain and between nociceptive and neuropathic pain if we are to understand both the advantages and the drawbacks of this class of drugs (Arnér and Meyerson 1988; Fields 1988). The patient with acute pain can be expected to resume normal activities when the injury heals and the pain stops. The role of the physician is to hasten healing and to provide temporary pain relief. Opiate drugs are the mainstay of this strategy; they have demonstrated efficacy and little or no risk for abuse or addiction when used to treat acute pain.

Research with chronic pain patients has consistently shown that just alleviating the symptom of pain is not sufficient. Recovery of good health requires the restoration of function, the relearning of skills and attitudes, and the facilitation of social interactions. Desired outcomes in the management of chronic pain include reduced pain, improved functioning, decreased health care consumption, return to work, patient satisfaction, and better quality of life. Opiates alone will often fail to achieve these more comprehensive outcome goals. Their side effects can contribute to continued disability, and the pain may not be adequately alleviated. Clinicians thus continue to seek a new opioid, or a new drug delivery system, or a new understanding of the patient-drug relationship that will solve the all too common clinical problems associated with prolonged opiate usage. Are alteration of mood and the risk of addiction an inherent and inescapable property of molecules that bind to μ-opioid receptors? Perhaps opioids can be designed and synthesized that do not have dose-limiting side effects.

Pain relief has certainly occurred in many patients who receive opiates, as it has in chronic pain patients treated with antiepileptics, tricyclic antidepressants, nonsteroidal anti-inflammatory drugs, and topical local anesthetics (Rowbotham 1999). However, repeated studies have shown that pain is reduced by about one-third, on average, for these chronic pain patients, *no matter what the disease or the drug*. Thus, two-thirds of the pain problem still lies outside the realm of our current pharmaceutical expertise. We must always ask the question: "Are opioids the best therapy that can be utilized today for this patient?" (Harden 2002). We should also ask, in the wise words of Santayana: "What can we learn from the lessons of history so that we are not destined to repeat them?"

REFERENCES

Arnér S, Meyerson BA. Lack of analgesia effect of opioids on neuropathic and idiopathic forms of pain. *Pain* 1988; 33:11–23.
Davenport-Hines R. *The Pursuit of Oblivion: A Global History of Narcotics*. New York: W.W. Norton, 2002.
De Quincey T. *Confessions of an Opium Eater*. New York: Viking Penguin, 1971.
Eldridge WB. *Narcotics and the Law*. Chicago: University of Chicago Press, 1962.
Fields HL. Can opiates relieve neuropathic pain? *Pain* 1988; 35:365.
Foley K. The treatment of cancer pain. *N Engl J Med* 1985; 313:84–95.
Harden RN. Chronic opioid therapy: another reappraisal. *APS Bulletin* 2002; 12:1–12.
Holmes OW. *Medical Essays of Oliver Wendell Holmes*. Birmingham: Classics of Medicine Library, 1961.
Huxley A. *The Doors of Perception*. New York: Harper and Row, 1963.
King R. *The Drug Hang Up*. New York: W.W. Norton, 1972.
Rowbotham MC. The debate over opioids and neuropathic pain. In: Kalso E, McQuay HJ, Wiesenfeld-Hallin Z (Eds). *Opioid Sensitivity of Chronic Noncancer Pain*, Progress in Pain Research and Management, Vol. 14. Seattle: IASP Press, 1999, pp 307–317.
Turner J, Calsyn DA, Fordyce WE, Ready LB. Drug utilization patterns in chronic pain patients. *Pain* 1982; 12:357–363.

Correspondence to: John D. Loeser, MD, Department of Neurological Surgery, University of Washington, Box 356470, Seattle, WA 98195, USA. Tel: 206-543-3570; Fax: 206-543-8315; email: jdloeser@u.washington.edu.

Opioids and Pain Relief: A Historical Perspective,
Progress in Pain Research and Management, Vol.
25, edited by Marcia L. Meldrum, IASP Press,
Seattle, © 2003.

2

To Market, to Market: The Theory and Practice of Opiates in the Middle Ages

Walton O. Schalick III

Departments of Pediatrics and History, Washington University in St. Louis, St. Louis, Missouri, USA

Given the interdisciplinary nature of the chapters in this volume, I will try to bridge a chasm—one that often bars discussion of ancient or medieval medicine in a more modern medical forum—that of efficacy. During the week of the conference on opioids on which this volume is based, National Public Radio's *Talk of the Nation* broadcast a show on birth control that opened with a segment on medieval prescriptions for preventing pregnancy. Included were such appealing ingredients as mule earwax, the testicles of a weasel, and the bones of the right side of a cat. The discordant humor was palpable. Similarly, when I lecture to a lay audience about medicine in the Middle Ages, the most frequent question is: "Well, did the therapies work?" The unspoken corollary is: "If the therapies did not work, why did these so-called physicians continue to use such bizarre remedies?" The power of retrospection is a remarkably potent blinder to the verities of history. Blinders similarly mask our own therapeutic foibles.

A recent study by Moseley and colleagues (2002) used sham arthroscopic surgery to debunk the efficacy of this modern therapy for osteoarthritis. A historian of the year 3003 looking back upon our practices in the 1990s might readily ask why we continued to use such an intrusive procedure if it did not "really" work.

The use of opium in the Middle Ages is the near antithesis of the stereotypical medical remedy of that age, such as those mentioned above. We "know" it works from ample scientific and experiential evidence today, but did medieval physicians use opiates and recognize their value? The answers are relevant at a variety of levels. First, Arabic traders probably introduced opium to much of Europe during the 13th century. How Europeans of this age perceived opium is thus important to our appreciation of its history, particularly because by the 16th century its abuse potential had become a matter of medical commentary (Brownstein 1993). Second, the university was born in Europe during the 13th century, and this institution continues to shape the landscape of our contemporary medical world. How the earliest university scholars approached a potentially sensitive subject like opiates can reveal much about the nature of our contiguous medical tradition. Finally, histories of opiate use during the high and late Middle Ages are exceedingly scarce (Seefelder 1987; Bonica 1990; Booth 1996). I hope this chapter may serve as a springboard for future investigation. As the 2002 conference focused on opiates rather than on pain itself, I will leave consideration of pain in the Middle Ages largely to another work (W.O. Schalick, unpublished manuscript).

The questions I have raised begin with the notion of efficacy and lead ineluctably toward social contexts of medieval medical practice. As modern observers looking back to an example from history, we may divide the issue into two parts: availability of a therapy that today has proven effectiveness in a given clinical setting, and historical use of that therapy in an appropriate medical setting. Pharmacopoeia dating to at least the third millennium before the Common Era included mention of opium. We know that the drug was distilled or prepared in sufficiently pure concentrations to generate physiological effects (Seefelder 1987). Today, we observe that those effects include the narcotic, sedative, euphoric, and hypnotic. In premodern times, observers remarked upon all these effects with varying degrees of clarity.

Did premodern physicians use opium and opioids in appropriate clinical settings? Several scholars have taken a historically nuanced approach to the analysis of references to potentially active pharmaceuticals in premodern texts (Majno 1991; Riddle 1992; Cameron 1993; Holland 1996; van Arsdall 2002). Collectively, they suggest that ancient and medieval physicians did not ignore their own experience in their practice, despite the lack of an "evidence base," but rather were able witnesses of overtly active drugs. Honey, wine, myrrh, and cupric salts (derived from preparing drug recipes in copper kettles) all have verifiable beneficial effects. Nevertheless, if a premodern physician suggested using a remedy in an appropriate setting along with another medication that could have been helpful in a modern sense, does the historian have sufficient evidence to judge the therapy as rational according to our own standards? The difficulty of making such a judgment is accentuated by the tendency of premodern physicians to list more than one remedy for a given condition. Some of these remedies are now known to be physiologically effective while others are considered ineffective.

In 1998, Prioreschi and his colleagues proposed a concise, retrospective measure of this characteristic of historic practice: the efficacy quotient (EQ). They acknowledged that many scholars today have presumed that a drug with a verifiable physiological effect must have been used in premodern times for that purpose, and they sought to test the presumption as a hypothesis. Their analysis began with a mathematical formula balancing the number of times a drug was used correctly, in a modern sense, with the number of times it was used incorrectly. They named the resulting heuristic metric the EQ. An EQ of 1 indicates that the prescriber used a drug as often for inappropriate conditions as for appropriate ones. Consequently, even though the drug has a bona fide effect, the premodern author did not always use it in appropriate settings or used ineffective remedies just as frequently or more often. Prioreschi and his colleagues examined 150 uses of opiates noted in the *Hippocratic Corpus* and calculated an EQ of 1.08 with a range of error of 0.49–1.54. Given that the range of error included an EQ of 1, it appears that Hippocratic physicians used opiates in an indiscriminate fashion, despite their physiological effect.

Several challenges mitigate against accepting this heuristic at face value. The challenges are even greater when applying the EQ to medieval pharmacology. Compound medicines had become more popular by the 13th and 14th centuries, so choosing a given compound drug for a particular condition based on one ingredient alone became all the harder. Furthermore, any single text prescribed fewer pharmaceuticals of a given class; hence the "*n*" for an EQ of a specific medieval author would be so small as to make the metric almost pointless for that author.

If the EQ is so fraught with challenges for examining the use of opiates in the Middle Ages, how can we better understand the medieval physician's choice of these agents? Surveying the medieval use of opiates yields three conclusions: (1) Medieval physicians acknowledged today's physiological effects of opiates: analgesia, somnolence, constipation, and mood alteration (Al-Fallouji 1997). (2) These same physicians recommended the use of opiates in clinical settings that today we consider physiologically appropriate (if not clinically so), for example, in cases of joint pain or severe headaches (Campbell and Colton 1960; Voigts and Hudson 1992; Isler et al. 1996). Marcellus, in the early fifth century, devoted 5% of a book on medicine to listing pharmaceutical remedies for headache, including one for a headache in a man, adolescent, or child occurring on the seventh day of the seventh month. His list included opium (Maximilianus 1916). One of his patients,

Libanius, praised Marcellus for curing his severe headaches (Thorndike 1923). In a Salernitan treatise of the 11th and 12th centuries, the herb *Papaver silvaticum*, a form of poppy, was listed as helping in *"emigraneum* or *dolor capatis,"* both terms for headaches (Howald and Sigerist 1927). (3) Medieval medical practitioners also frequently recommended opiates in settings that we would consider physiologically inappropriate, such as to dry up a runny nose or soothe a crying child (Pagel 1894; Alexandre-Bidon and Lett 1999; Ramoutsaki et al. 2002). Given the frequency of these latter uses of opiates, we must again ask why they were used for such variant complaints.

One answer lies not in the factual realm of modern science, but in the way medicine was practiced in the Middle Ages. Just as physicians today choose medications for reasons that may be more social than experimentally justified—for example, prescribing antibiotics to assuage the parents of a child with an earache, selecting therapies based on insurance pressures, or performing arthroscopies for osteoarthritis—so, too, did medieval physicians respond to and exert social influence in their approach to drugs. It is thus important to understand the place of these physicians within the medical marketplace and within society to better appreciate why and how they selected drugs.

THE EMERGING ROLES OF ACADEMICIANS AND APOTHECARIES

Before the advent of the university, European medicine was broadly practiced by figures who may be generally termed " medical practitioners," as opposed to the later academic "physician." No English terminology easily distinguishes the different kinds of medical workers in the Middle Ages. Terms such as "doctor," from the Latin *doctore* meaning "to teach," and "physician," from the Latin *physicus* meaning both "physical scientist" and "physician," are significantly entangled in their etymology. Curiously, the English meanings of these terms differ markedly from the meanings in other European languages (Bylebyl 1990). While "medical practitioner" is both cumbersome and elusive, it may help the modern reader follow the subsequent discussion. (Where the term "doctor" appears below, it includes both "physicians" and "medical practitioners.") Often trained in some more or less codified apprenticeship, these practitioners could be either itinerant or static in their work. Early medieval medical practitioners collected and dispensed herbs, performed rudimentary surgeries, cared for common nonsurgical diseases, and sometimes taught others while creating new medical knowledge. Certainly some practitioners, either by skill or chance, concentrated their activities in a particular category, such as setting broken bones or cutting for bladder stones. By and large, however, medical activity was more general before the advent of the universities (Siraisi 1990; Schalick 1997).

The 11th and 12th centuries saw the rise of increasingly settled schools, centered in cathedrals and towns. The medical school at Salerno became particularly successful, but was soon overshadowed by the formation of the first universities, in Paris and Bologna, at the end of the 12th and beginning of the 13th centuries.

 Precisely what caused the separation of one medical activity from another is unclear. Nevertheless, by the 12th century, we find references to surgeons and "internists," for lack of a better word, and by the 13th century, in the north of Europe at least, university-trained physicians vociferously proclaimed their difference from lay surgeons, generalized medical practitioners, and herb sellers. Moreover, these "sour word-specialists," as one contemporary poet described them, asserted their supremacy in the medical world, appointing themselves to the pinnacle of the pyramid of medieval medicine (Rutebeuf 1990; Jacquart 1998).

Characters such as Jean de Saint-Amand (c. 1240–1303), one of the first professors of the University of Paris medical faculty, in essence formed a guild of textualist-physicians who specialized in interpreting the growing number of ancient medical texts then being translated from Greek and Arabic. With the translations came innumerable linguistically and philosophically nuanced problems needing resolution (García-Ballester 1998). Among the most important of these translations were the works of Avicenna (980–1037), the great Persian physician, philosopher, and mathematician. Saint-Amand was the first professor to comment upon Avicenna. He came from the region that is now Belgium, but presumably studied medicine in Paris and gradually rose to a faculty position. He has left us over one million words about medical education and medical pharmacology (Schalick 1997).

Saint-Amand was particularly adept at assimilating these new texts and culling pharmacological information. In response to the clamors of students spending wakeful nights sifting through large medical volumes, he adapted the recently invented concordance to present this new information to students and other physicians. Saint-Amand and his colleagues suggested that their refined knowledge was the only source for appropriately directing medical care.

The university physician did not exist in a vacuum, however, for with his emergence came the more specialized surgeon and drug seller. Apothecaries, for example, derived their name from the fixed shop, *apotheca,* which became their retail venue. They sold both local and exotic remedies, and typically other wares as well, but some became particularly known for their medical products. We know little about their activities during this period because the guild and financial records from northern Europe were lost over the ages. Nevertheless, from a variety of medical, lay, and fictional sources, we may deduce that the drug sellers made their living in a culture that was mostly oral rather than textual (Schalick 1997).

Interestingly, the field of drug selling also became subspecialized by the late 13th and early 14th centuries. In tax data from Paris, I have identified three categories of drug sellers—*épicers* (pharmacists), *mires* (medical practitioners), and *herbiers* (herbalists). Rough information culled from the tax data suggests that the *épicers* were the most numerous and their relative incomes higher compared to sellers in the other groups (based on the assumption that the more tax they paid, the greater their income). The itinerant *mires* and *herbiers* fared less well (Schalick 1997).

Consequently, a subpyramid of drug practitioners is notable in 13th- and 14th-century Paris, with the pharmacist above the medical practitioner, who was in turn above the herbalist. Such differentiation implies that the medical marketplace encompassed dramatic competitive forces that split practitioners into increasingly specialized fields, not unlike the gross economic forces operating today.

ROYAL REGULATIONS

Little work has been done to characterize the 13th- and 14th-century Parisian patient. However, one variety of patient, the royalty, played an important role in defining the Parisian marketplace. As the century progressed, the university settled in buildings on the Left Bank not far from one of the most concentrated centers of apothecary shops, the Petit Pont. University medical masters walking that bridge were constantly accosted by merchants selling concoctions for medicinal purposes, opiates and laxatives among them. Using their increasing influence at the court of Paris, the university masters applied to the kings of France for stricter medical regulation.

In a sequence of ordinances from the beginning of the 14th century, the French kings progressively regulated pharmaceutical practice. In response to arguments made by the university physicians, the court ruled that certain kinds of drugs could only be dispensed under the direction of the physicians or their agents. In particular, laxatives and opiates were targeted for careful regulation from 1311 to 1353 (de Laurière and Secousse 1723 and 1729). The royal ordinances repeatedly mentioned these two kinds of remedies, perhaps because of several deaths from improper use.

The Parisian medical marketplace at the turn of the 14th century thus embraced two spheres of activity. One was the sphere of the university physician, his authority buttressed with texts and theory derived from the new translations. The other encompassed the lay activity of the various drug sellers, surgeons, and medical practitioners, which was highly practical in its orientation, orally based in its knowledge structure, and more or less itinerant in its setting. These spheres were usually distinct in their boundaries and frequently antagonistic toward each other, often diametrically so. In the interaction of these two spheres we can find one reason for the medical interest in opiates.

The medical regulations to which I refer appeared in two tandem streams of events during the time of Saint-Amand's work. First, the university medical faculty promulgated two pronouncements about the practice of medicine. The first, in 1271, included a long list of injunctions, among them a specific clause limiting pharmaceutical practice, with a focus on laxative medicines in particular. Certain medicines could be dispensed free of a physician's supervision, for example, *sucura rosata, dragia communis,* and *aqua rosacea,* drugs of no evident physiological activity. Following these medicines, in increasing order of concern to the faculty, were laxative medicines and then alterative or comforting drugs (Denifle and Chaelain 1889, t. I). In 1322, the university physicians again announced their regulatory desires, but they included opiates along with laxatives as drugs of concern (Denifle and Chaelain 1889, t. II). This reiteration of their previous stance came in the middle of the series of edicts by the kings of France; in that juxtaposition we may detect the insinuation of faculty interests into the royal court.

The royal ordinances began in 1311, in response to "a great complaint from several directions" regarding the "frauds and tricks of spice vendors and of their improprieties in weighing wares" (de Laurière and Secousse 1723, t. I). The apothecaries were enjoined to use a newer and more closely monitored measuring system and were also required to have approved scales. The king exempted physicians and surgeons, allowing them to use an older system of weights with fewer regulations. Curiously, only one month previously, the king had centralized control of all surgical practice in the hands of his royal surgeon. Simultaneously, he praised the university faculty for their avid pursuit of medical science, calling them the "Samaritans" who bathed the ignorant in a river of learning (Nicaise 1902). The pyramid of medical authority was becoming concrete.

In a 1336 royal ordinance, the new king, Philip VI, stipulated that apothecaries must swear loyalty to these praiseworthy physicians, whose specialized knowledge directed the best medical practices. This edict singled out opiates and laxatives for careful monitoring by the physicians because their use posed the danger of death (de Laurière and Secousse 1729, t. II). Finally, in 1352, a royal ordinance again listed opiates, and also six laxatives, as needing the attention of medical authorities (Denifle and Chaelain 1889, t. III). In a repetitive and increasingly specific fashion, opiate use came under the regulatory mandate of the learned medical faculty.

I would assert that such a conclusion had practical ramifications for the pharmaceutical marketplace. In particular, the 1322 pronouncement of the medical faculty stipulated that:

> When the aforementioned apothecaries dispense any recipes from (the *Antidotary of*) *Nicholas* [the textbook for pharmaceutical preparation standardized by the medical faculty and by Jean de Saint-Amand, in particular] be they laxatives or opiates, they should not prepare them until they have shown them to the aforementioned dean [of the Medical Faculty] …, and when they have prepared them, they should write upon them the month when they were made, and if they have become corrupted, one should dispose of them. (Denifle and Chaelain 1889, t. II)

The age of the drug preparation was thus crucial and had to be documented. It is also notable that the *Antidotary of Nicholas* was the benchmark for preparing drugs (Goltz 1976). This text, originally written in the south of Europe at the highly practical medical school of Salerno, was one of a handful of Salernitan texts absorbed into the highly theoretical curriculum of the northern medical universities. Saint-Amand's commentary and correction of that text were among his most lasting contemporary legacies (Saint-Amand 1549).

OPIATE THEORY AND THE MARKETPLACE

Why were the dangers of opiates and laxatives, and the age of these medications, becoming royal concerns? I have argued elsewhere that during the 13th century, academic physicians were influenced in their interpretation of traditional medical practice by the waves of translations of Hippocrates, Galen, and Avicenna. In the case of laxatives, Saint-Amand dwelled especially on the dangerous side effects of their use, and accused lay practitioners of ignorance about the theory of pharmaceuticals. A comparison of Saint-Amand's descriptions of laxatives and their dangers with those of three other 13th-century medical authors, reveals that Saint-Amand was three times more likely to describe side effects than were the other authors. Simultaneously, medical authorities also began to see danger in opiate use (Schalick 1997).

Roger Bacon, an academician who died in 1294, spent several years in Paris and wrote a treatise entitled the "Errors of Doctors." Among their many frailties, Bacon noted:

The ordinary doctor knows nothing about simple drugs, but entrusts himself to ignorant apothecaries, concerning whom it is agreed by these doctors themselves that they have no other purpose but to deceive. The apothecaries cheat them in various ways. One is in the price of drugs, and as a result the patients are overcharged. Likewise in the quality of the drugs: first, because they give old drugs for new ones; [or] one thing [is substituted] instead of another, for example an artificial bone instead of the bone of the stag's heart, ... and so on indefinitely ... (Wellborn 1932)

Regarding opiates, Bacon noted two cardinal deficiencies in doctors:

[They are ignorant of] the relation between the quantity of noxious drugs and the body, e.g., scammony and opium, nor is the method of giving them known, nor in what quantities, nor what quantity for which condition or age; therefore death follows, or frequently a bodily insensibility, and various diseases, and through scammony a man may incur dysentery and death, and through opium, frenzy. (Wellborn 1932)

Laxatives could cause dehydration and death, but opium provoked a loss of a self-control, a "frenzy." For Bacon, the doctor's second deficiency with respect to opiates was more theoretical:

[The important element] ... is in the fermentation of drugs; [according to Avicenna] duration is the key, but there is no theory [to support this principle], except that an opiate drug should not be brought forth before the end of six months. ... But time alone does not cause fermentation unless some other device is used along with it, because neither the narcotic in an opiate nor *diagredium* [the active ingredient] in a laxative is fermented with its simples unless it is reduced to one single substance. To work one needs three things—time, good mixing and dissolution of the poisonous material—and this is the secret of secrets of which all the common doctors are ignorant. (Wellborn 1932)

In Bacon's view, the poisonous root of opiates, and laxatives, had to be eradicated before they could be used safely, but physicians had no theoretical system to guide them.

Roger Baron (fl. 1240–1250), an enigmatic physician in Paris, attested to the extent of the consequent therapeutic paralysis in the mid-13th century.

He devoted a long section of his work, *On Medications,* to laxatives (Baron 1326). The section begins:

> Since, however, the medical arts are of two parts, namely theory and practice, and they are believed to be integral in care, practice sets its entire utility in their combination. Indeed the attention of practice is twined around the rules and orderly arrangements of medicinal laxatives and the coinciding exhibitions of opiates all the more strongly and closely. Whence for all practical use that laxative medicine ought to be preferred which is weak and debilitated rather than robust and strong in any quantity and substance, at any time and for any cause. (Baron 1326)

This passage is important in showing that, just prior to Saint-Amand's work, opiates and laxatives were treated largely as practical rather than theoretical matters, and that practitioners were so worried about their use and so unsure of how to control the active ingredients and their side effects that they preferred less potent concoctions.

The danger of such medications in the wrong hands was not lost on academic practitioners of that time, as seen in a report of an apothecary's mistake. Bernard de Gordon, writing in the early 14th century at the University of Montpellier, tells the story of an apothecary who sold a compound medicine, theriac, that included opium and more than 60 other ingredients. Unfortunately, the apothecary left some of the drug on his thumbnail. After picking at his nose, he changed color and lost consciousness. Bernard was summoned. He realized that the apothecary had used too much theriac and gave the patient an emetic followed by a dose of the appropriate amount of theriac (Demaitre 1980; Thomasset 1994). The perceptive physician had to be cautious. The responsible physician was obligated to restrict the practice of careless practitioners.

In the preface of his *Areolae*, a textbook on simples (medications that worked without being mixed with other ingredients) probably written in the 1290s, Saint-Amand described the purpose of his work:

> Thus said Galen …, "It is not possible for a man to receive well a compound medicine (or) use, according to the manner he ought, a medicine made by another for him, and competently compound it, unless he knows the virtues of simple medicines." The cause of this, however, is (that in) the mixture and fermentation of simple medicines comes a certain form in the compound and this form cannot be exactly appreciated, unless we understand the virtue, the substance and complexion of simple medicines and their appropriate doses. (Pagel 1893)

The root element of a drug, the "form in the compound," which so aroused Bacon's theoretical and Baron's practical concern about opiates, became a central focus of Saint-Amand's academic texts. In essence, the individual actions of component medicines were important for Saint-Amand, and opiates were a necessary topic of instruction at the university (McVaugh 1965, 1975). In describing how critical it was for a physician to understand the diseases he treated, Saint-Amand highlighted the use of opiates as therapy for severe pain. "First we act against the substance of the pain by mortifying and restoring the stunned member through narcotics or opium, *mandragora*, and others so that the member does not sense [the pain]" (Saint-Amand 1549). Pragmatically, Saint-Amand was moving the playing field of pharmaceuticals from the place of practice to that of theory, and opiates were important players on that field.

For Saint-Amand, the importance of opiates and laxatives lay in their contrary effects. A laxative caused a gastrointestinal flux, which, by the metaphorical medical theory of the time, meant that it promoted a general flux in the body. Opiates, in contrast, had a constipative effect. Thus, an opiate taken in advance of a laxative could minimize the consequent, life-threatening diarrhea.

> Likewise, the doctor ought to take care to expunge the harmful effects from a drug. Thus he ought first to give [opium]; it cancels out the danger [of the laxatives], ... but the laxative is an "imperfect opposite" of an opiate, because the drug ages and causes many other side effects, while opium causes many salubrious effects—it comforts, consumes matter and constrains members. It is used as a contrastive agent by the common practitioner (Pagel 1893).

According to Walter of Agilon, a somewhat shadowy scholar whose work was nonetheless cited by Saint-Amand's contemporary Arnau de Vilanova (d. 1311), opiates had three "virtues:" (1) they arrested the humoral flow into a part of the body, (2) they strengthened the body part nurtured by that flow, and (3) they consumed the flow of humors. Some compounded opiates were administered before a laxative, such as *dyamoron* (a mixture of boiled rose, licorice, and poppy), thus stopping the supposed flow of humor to the throat muscles; others, such as *Aurea Alexandrine,* were given after laxatives, in this case as a gargle for head ailments, among others. Especially in fevers, opium-based drugs were to be used cautiously (Sheahan 1938; Agilius 13**). According to humoral theory, which used descriptions of qualities such as hot, cold, wet, and dry, opium could be considered a "cold" medicine whose action could cool the heat of painful diseases (Saint-Amand 1549).

The challenges of treating patients with multiple agents, in particular when given in combination, as in the compound medicines above, also concerned Saint-Amand. For example, in his commentary on the authoritative *Antidotary of Nicholas*, which extolled that text as the final word on understanding simple and compound remedies, Saint-Amand observed that "it is not possible that a man understand compound medicine, unless he first understands simple medicines, thus Nicholas made a determination on the understanding of compound medicines: 'First, we ought to consider simple medicines …'" (Saint-Amand 1549). The *Antidotary* became the regulatory benchmark for practicing pharmacists in Paris after the 1353 ordinance, as the king now demanded they keep a corrected copy of this text available at all times. The corrections had to be certified by the medical faculty, which used Saint-Amand's treatise as its "bible."

The nuances of using these medications, as Bacon complained earlier, were emphasized in a focus on the age of opiate preparations in apothecary shops. From a regulatory standpoint, the king in May 1336 requested that the "Masters (of university medicine) examine medical laxatives, and opiates, which are stored for a long time, before they become compounded, and ascertain that they are good and fresh and not corrupted" (de Laurière and Secousse 1729, t. II).

Certainly, both these demands were aimed, in part, at keeping "fresh" medicines on the shelves of the apothecaries. In this sense, the 1336 ordinance identified a contemporary problem: some drugs sold by apothecaries were not active (i.e., not fresh). The inactivation could arise from processes that the ordinance did not describe, but the concern with time was new, as compared to the 1271 faculty statute or the preceding royal ordinances. The king's mandate now recognized that opiates were stored for longer periods, presumably to become active, as Bacon described above. This necessary aging also was not a cause of opiates becoming inactive, but it was a novel description in the evolving regulatory language.

Such a new element most likely arose from Avicenna's notion of time-dependent "fermentation" and the adaptations made to the concept by physicians such as Saint-Amand. Not surprisingly, Saint-Amand wrote about the variable use of opiates of different ages. In his *Expositio*, he looked at whether new or old mixed opiates were better and concluded that it depended on the condition the physician was trying to cure (Saint-Amand 1549). Expert knowledge and experience were critical to the proper use of these drugs. The university physician had that expertise.

THE MORE THINGS CHANGE ...

Recent research has emphasized the religious, philosophical, and intellectual underpinnings of scholastic medical arguments over pain (Cohen 1995, 2000; Salmón 1996, 2000; Rey 1998). Yet, the treatment of pain also played an important role in the "professional" life of medieval physicians. As an early critic of lay medicine noted:

> Other monks, becoming cognizant of their inadequate grounding in philosophy, have become medical students. Then suddenly, in the twinkling of an eye, they have blossomed forth as the same kind of physicians that they had previously been Philosophers [i.e., ignorant]. Stocked with fallacious empirical rules they return after a brief interval to practice with sedulity what they learned. ... They are revered as omnipotent, because this is what they boast and promise. However, I have observed that there are two rules that they are more especially prone to recall and put into practice ... from Hippocrates ...: "Where there is indulgence, one ought not to labor." and "Take [your fee] while the patient is in pain." (McVaugh 1997)

Pain was certainly a feature of medieval life, just as it is of ours (Duby 1995). One explanation for why we have pain, which had greater *caché* in the Middle Ages than today, was the identification of the origin of pain in Eve's sin as described in Genesis 3:16 and 17. Religious beliefs, however, were not the only explanations. In the world of marketplace strategizing, the dangerous side effects of opiate use were an element added to the pharmocopoeic literature by elite, textually based physicians such as Saint-Amand; the result was a secularization of pain. Side effects, whether real or imagined from our point of view, became a market force that mandated control of prescriptions by experts such as Saint-Amand and his university colleagues.

In addition, university physicians wrote treatises about the dangers of laxatives and opiates, accentuating the importance of appropriately prescribing these medicines based on the knowledge derived from the new medical translations. Balancing these two medications allowed medical theoreticians to generate more elaborate ideas about the action of drugs on the body. Such new theories provided the basis of authority that enabled the royal courts to exert influence over all medical practice within the bounds of Paris.

When Saint-Amand endorsed the use of an opiate to dry up a runny nose, we should not summarily dismiss his action as that of a benighted physician working before the enlightenment of medical science (Pagel 1894).

Saint-Amand's decision was based on the place of opium within his own system of "rational" medicine, a system that was influenced by the functioning of medicine in society. Consequently, we might posit that patients with rhinorrhea demanded medicines that were seen both as powerful and as the subject of contemporary discussion. Opiates were certainly both.

While we lack direct evidence that such was the case, we do know that physicians complained about the untutored demands of their patients. One 14th-century doctor trained in treating patients with phlebotomy or by diet and other regimen changes, complained that "Many patients in these modern days are particularly impatient" for more rapid cures than could be affected by regimens (Getz 1992). A patient's demand of opiates for rhinorrhea is no more difficult to appreciate than today's patients' demands for antibiotics to treat viral ear infections or for arthroscopy to help their osteoarthritis. Clearly the professional and social perceptions of opiates, laxatives, and similar drugs in regulation, bargaining, and practice, and in theory, need to be added to our "compounded" explanation for premodern pharmaceutical use.

Several other chapters in this volume highlight modern regulation of opiates, concern for their dangerous side effects, and the search for medications to mitigate that danger. In the vein of the time-honored French expression, *"plus ça change, plus ça reste le même"* ("the more things change, the more they stay the same"), we hear these same concerns in 13th- and 14th-century Paris. While we observe similarity in change, we also encounter noteworthy variation. For medieval physicians and laity, opiates held significant meaning beyond our contemporary notions of physiological efficacy. Effects of these drugs, "real" or otherwise, extended well into the boundaries of social control and economics long before addiction and abuse became a focus of social debate.

ACKNOWLEDGMENTS

Support for this project came in part from a Robert Wood Johnson Generalist Faculty Scholar Award. I am grateful to Dr. Marcia Meldrum for the invitation to participate and for scholarly insights along the way. I also thank the participants in the UCLA/John C. Liebeskind Collection's second History of Pain Symposium, the History and Philosophy of Science Brown Bag Group at Washington University, Professor Mark Gregory Pegg, Natasha Winters Schalick, and an outside reviewer for comments.

REFERENCES

Agilius G, 13**. Liber de dosi medicinarum. *Erfurt Q* 185, fo. 38r–44v.

Alexandre-Bidon D, Lett D. *Children in the Middle Ages, Fifth–Fifteenth Centuries.* Gladding J (Trans). Notre Dame, IN: University of Notre Dame Press, 1999.

Al-Fallouji M. Arabs were skilled in anaesthesia. *BMJ* 1997; 314:1128.

Baron R. Practica. In: *Paneth Codex.* Yale Medical Library, 1326, fo. 510–584.

Bonica JJ. *The Management of Pain,* 2nd ed., Vol. 1. Philadelphia: Lea & Febiger, 1990.

Booth M. *Opium: A History.* New York: St. Martin's Griffin, 1996.

Brownstein MJ. A brief history of opiates, opioid peptides, and opioid receptors. *Proc Natl Acad Sci USA* 1993; 90:5391–5393.

Bylebyl JJ. The medical meaning of *Physica.* In: McVaugh MR, Siraisi NG (Eds). Renaissance medical learning: evolution of a tradition. *Osiris* 1990; 6:16–41.

Cameron ML. *Anglo-Saxon Medicine.* Cambridge Studies in Anglo-Saxon England, Vol. 7. Cambridge: Cambridge University Press, 1993.

Campbell E, Colton J. *The Surgery of Theodoric, ca. A.D. 1267.* New York: Appleton-Century-Crofts, 1960.

Cohen E. Towards a history of European physical sensibility: pain in the later middle ages. *Science in Context* 1995: 8:47–74.

Cohen E. The animated pain of the body. *Am Hist Rev* 2000; 105:36–68.

de Laurière EJ, Secousse DF (Eds). *Ordonnances des roys de France, 1723 and 1729.* Ts. I–II. Paris: L'Imprimerie Royale.

Demaitre LE. *Doctor Bernard of Gordon: Professor and Practitioner.* Toronto: Pontifical Institute of Mediaeval Studies, 1980.

Denifle H, Chaelain A (Eds). *Chartularium Universitatis Parisiensis.* Ts. I–II. Paris: Imprimerie, 1889.

Duby G. Réflexions sur la douleur physique au moyen age. In: Levy G (Ed). *La Douleur 'Audela des Maux'.* Paris: Editions des Archives Contemporaines, 1995, pp 71–79.

García-Ballester L. The 'New Galen': a challenge to Latin Galenism in thirteenth-century Montpellier. In: Fischer K-D, Nickel D, Potter P (Eds). *Text and Tradition: Studies in Ancient Medicine and Its Transmission.* Leiden: Brill, 1998, 55–84.

Getz FM. The Faculty of Medicine before 1500. In: Catto JI, Evans E (Eds). *Late Medieval Oxford,* The History of the University of Oxford, Vol. II. Oxford: Clarendon Press, 1992, pp 373–405.

Goltz D. *Mittelalterliche Pharmazie und Medizin: Dargestellt an Geschichte und Inhalt des Antidotarium Nicolai: Mit ein Nachdruck der Druckfassung von 1471.* Veröffentlichungen der Internationalen Gesellschaft für Geschichte der Pharmazie e.V., Vol. 44. Stuttgart: Wissenschaftliche Verlagsgesellschaft MBH, 1976.

Holland BK. *Prospecting for Drugs in Ancient and Medieval European Texts: A Scientific Approach.* Amsterdam: Harwood, 1996.

Howald E, Sigerist H. *Antonii Musae De herba vettonica liber, Pseudoapulei Herbarius, Anonymi De taxone liber, (et) Sexti Placiti Liber medicinae ex animalibus.* Leipzig: B.G. Teubner, 1927.

Isler H, Hasenfratz H, O'Neill T. A sixth-century Irish headache cure and its use in a south German monastery. *Cephalgia* 1996; 16:536–540.

Jacquart D. *La médecine médiévale dans le cadre Parisien.* Paris: Fayard, 1998.

Majno G. *The Healing Hand: Man and Wound in the Ancient World.* Cambridge: Harvard University Press, 1991.

Maximilianus N (Ed). *Marcelli de medicamentis liber,* Corpus Medicorum Latinorum, Vol. 5. Leipzig: Teubner, 1916.

McVaugh MR. The mediaeval theory of compound medicines. PhD dissertation, Princeton University, 1965.

McVaugh MR. Introduction. In: McVaugh MR (Ed). *Arnaldi de Villanova Opera Medical Omnia*, t. II. Granada: University of Barcelona, 1975.

McVaugh MR. Bedside manners in the Middle Ages. *Bull Hist Med* 1997; 71:201–223.

Moseley JB, O'Malley K, Petersen NJ, et al. A controlled trial of arthroscopic surgery for osteoarthritis of the knee. *N Engl J Med* 2002; 347:81–88.

Nicaise V. Chirurgiens et barbiers aux XIIIᵉ et XIVᵉ siècles. *Bull Soc Française Hist Med* 1902; 442–462.

Pagel J. *Die Areolae des Johannes de Sancto Amando (13. Jahrhundert)*. Berlin: Georg Reimer, 1893.

Pagel JL. *Die Concordanciae des Johannes de Sancto Amando*. Berlin: Georg Reimer, 1894.

Prioreschi P, Heaney RP, Brehm E. A quantitative assessment of ancient therapeutics: poppy and pain in the Hippocratic Corpus. *Med Hypotheses* 1998; 51:325–331.

Ramoutsaki IA, Dimitriou H, Kalmanti M. Management of childhood diseases in the Byzantine Period: I. Analgesia. *Pediatr Int* 2002; 44:335–337.

Rey R. *The History of Pain*. Wallace TE, Cadden JA, Cadden SW (Trans). Cambridge: Harvard University Press, 1998.

Riddle JM. *Contraception and Abortion from the Ancient World to the Renaissance*. Cambridge, MA: Harvard University Press, 1992.

Rutebeuf. Li diz de l'erberie. In: Zink M (Ed, Trans). *Rutebeuf: Oeuvres completes*. T. II. Paris: Classiques Garnier, 1990, pp 240–251.

Saint-Amand J. Expositio super Antidotarium Nicolai. In: *Mesue et omnia quae cum eo imprimi*. Venice: Iuntas, 1549.

Salmón F. Academic discourse and pain in medical scholasticism (thirteenth-fourteenth centuries). In: Kottek SS, García-Ballester L (Eds). *Medicine and Medical Ethics in Medieval and Early Modern Spain: An Intercultural Approach*. Jerusalem: Magnes Press, 1996, pp 136–153.

Salmón F. Pain and the medieval physician. *Am Pain Soc Bull* 2000; 10:3.

Schalick WO. *Add One Part Pharmacy to One Part Surgery and One Part Medicine: Jean de Saint-Amand and the Development of Medical Pharmacology in Thirteenth-Century Paris*. Ann Arbor: UMI, 1997.

Seefelder M. *Opium: Eine Kulturgeschichte*. Frankfurt: Athenäum, 1987.

Sheahan S. An Irish version of Gaulterus de dosibus. PhD dissertation, Catholic University of America, 1938.

Siraisi NG. *Medieval & Early Renaissance Medicine: An Introduction to Knowledge and Practice*. Chicago: Chicago University Press, 1990.

Thomasset C. Bernard de Gordon: L'extraction des corps étrangers accidentellement introduits dans l'oreille. In: *Comprendre et maîtriser la nature au moyen age: Mélanges d'histoire des sciences offerts à Guy Beaujouan*. Geneva: Librairie Droz, 1994, pp 351–364.

Thorndike L. *A History of Magic and Experimental Science*, Vol. I. New York: Columbia University Press, 1923.

van Arsdall A. *Medieval Herbal Remedies: The Old English Herbarium and Anglo-Saxon Medicine*. London: Routledge, 2002.

Voigts LE, Hudson RP. A drynke þat men callen dwale to make a man to slepe whyle men kerven him: a surgical anesthetic from late medieval England. In: Campbell S, et al. (Eds). *Health, Disease and Healing in Medieval Culture*. New York: St. Martin's Press, 1992, pp 34–56.

Wellborn MC. The errors of the doctors according to Friar Roger Bacon of the Minor Order. *Isis* 1932, pp 26–62.

Correspondence to: Walton O. Schalick, III, MD, PhD, Department of Pediatrics, 5S20, Box 8116, Children's Hospital, Washington University, One Children's Place, St. Louis, MO 63110, USA. Email: schalick_w@kids.wustl.edu.

Opioids and Pain Relief: A Historical Perspective,
Progress in Pain Research and Management, Vol.
25, edited by Marcia L. Meldrum, IASP Press,
Seattle, © 2003.

3

"The Grandest Badge of His Art": Three Victorian Doctors, Pain Relief, and the Art of Medicine

Martha Stoddard Holmes

*Department of Literature and Writing Studies, California State University,
San Marcos, California, USA*

A wealth of scholarship has examined the "death of pain" on both sides of the Atlantic after William Morton's successful public demonstration of surgical anesthesia with ether in 1846 (Pernick 1985; Rey 1998; Stanley 2003). But what happened to nonsurgical pain after 1846? This chapter approaches the question by examining the writings of three 19th-century doctors about cancer pain. These texts, written for other doctors and for the literate general public, articulate the practice of managing and sometimes relieving the pain of seriously ill and dying people in the context of medical advances in surgical pain relief that heightened the hope that relief might extend to all manner of painful human maladies. When these doctors describe what it means to take away the pain of illness when the illness itself cannot be cured, they are mindful that the pain of cancer and other serious illnesses persists against the backdrop of surgical pain's demise. The pain they are relieving, I suggest, gained new status after 1846.

The belief that "the object of extinguishing the sufferings of surgery will never again be lost sight of by the medical profession and the public" (Davus 1847) and the "remarkable perfection" (Anonymous 1847) of surgical anesthesia heralded a seductive discourse of success that may have made nonsurgical pain the subject of greater frustration and less cultural investment on the part of medical researchers. The triumph over one kind of pain, figuring a potential victory over illness and even death itself, may have made the care of those whose pain could not be relieved a source of medical conflict and even shame. Pain, then, was not transformed equally throughout medical practice, and not even in the context of surgery. One of Pernick's major contributions to the study of the history of pain relief was to explain that anesthesia itself was not applied openhandedly after 1846. It depended, among other things, on the patient's location on a "calculus of suffering" that assessed how much his or her pain merited relief. In addition, as letters to the *Lancet* in the late 1840s testify, many doctors were simply concerned about the dangers of surgical anesthesia (e.g., Anonymous 1847). At the same time, the three Victorian doctors discussed below all make the relief of pain not simply a facet of their profession but its centerpiece. The different status held by pain relief in each text—whether it is a physician's duty, "the grandest badge" of the physician's art, the hallmark of a good death, or the key to the mystery of curing cancer—indicates the particular nature of each doctor's response to the prospect of relieving the pain of incurable illness. I will also allude to the engaging minor thread of these doctors' use of litera- ture as a supplement to other modes of articulating what is often inarticulable, pain itself.

As well as bringing to light an area of the history of pain relief that has not been extensively studied, this chapter introduces readers to medical writers who in all but one case were well known in their lifetimes, remind- ing us that even in the decades after the success of surgical anesthesia, a rich if minor Victorian discourse of pain and palliative care persisted alongside the extensive discourse of surgical analgesia.

As a literature and cultural studies scholar, I bring several assumptions to this project that will help situate my line of reasoning. First, pain is a physiological, social, and imaginative event. Here, of course, I am standing on the capacious shoulders of current humanities scholars like Elaine Scarry (1985) and David Morris (1991), but also on those of moral philosophers like Adam Smith, whose *Theory of Moral Sentiments* (1907, first published in 1752) explores how difficult it is to imagine the pain of another person and considers what personal and social frames of reference we may invoke in order to attempt such an act of imagination. Second, how we imagine and represent pain and how pain is treated in a clinical setting are interdepen- dent, mutually informing activities. This is true whether we are patients, doctors, nurses, legislators, family members, or novelists. I am not arguing that pain is all in our imaginations, or that cultural constructions of pain, including patient accounts, supersede other registers of bodily experience, but simply that imagination and representation are inextricably in dialogue with other truths about pain. As a result, when people imagine pain, they imagine it in ways that are culturally and historically particular. Finally, I assume that the question of how Victorian doctors imagined pain after the successful use of surgical anesthesia can best be addressed by analyzing writing that places us in scenes of medical practice and theorizes pain relief as part of the art of medicine.

These three doctors in the last half of the 19th century, I will suggest, imagined pain and its relief partly in the contexts of the "death of pain" in 1846 and of the gradual erosion of religious and other objections to removing pain from surgery (and later, from childbirth). The territory in which they wrote included both the idea of pain as an experience with religious meaning and the idea of pain as a sign of physical pathology or even as pathology itself. As the century proceeded, other issues entered the landscape in which doctors imagined pain, including the rise of imaging technology and a series of new "cure" ideas that at times competed with pain-free surgery as the method of choice for treating cancer and other terminal diseases. Concerns about drug dependency and the specter of the "dope fiend" ultimately entered this landscape as well.

After 1846, the landscape in which doctors imagined and treated pain was a terrain where the pain of the dying was increasingly out of place, at odds with medicine imagined as a field of technological cures and miracles. Another such shift occurred in the 1880s, with the introduction of the germ theory of disease. The doctor-patient relationship around pain—drastically changed in many ways by surgical anesthesia (Pernick 1985)—was not changed to the same extent in the case of chronic and terminal illness. The cancer patient could be both conscious and visibly and audibly suffering; the pain might be managed, but often it could not be alleviated. Unlike a discrete surgical event, moreover, the pain of chronic or terminal illness had to be addressed again and again. Pain belonged to a different kind of medical practice, one devoted to the care of the variable human being, who, then as now, experiences physical and mental difficulties, suffers, ages, and dies.

Texts written by doctors who continued to emphasize care of the ill and dying negotiate that landscape. Morris (1998) asserts that contemporary undertreatment of pain stems in part from physicians' attitudes "in a chain of transmission reaching back almost ... to the time of Coleridge." These attitudes include a belief in a separation between the "real" of the visible lesion and the "unreal" of the pain and suffering of others, based on a medical mind-body dualism he locates in the time of Byron. The words of the Victorian doctors introduced below, however, suggest an alternate strand of medical history in which "caring when cure is impossible" is central to the doctor's role and both suffering and pain are objects for the caring doctor. The broad gestures of theorists like Foucault (1973), which document the disappearance of the patient's story in favor of the cataloging of symptoms, tend to bypass these real if minor strains of concern for compassionate care that remained after the advent of surgical anesthesia and the rise of various seductive and exciting narratives of cure. The writings of these doctors may be relevant to our own time, in which what can be imagined about the body through medical technologies continues to exceed our ability to work through the ethical issues technology raises, and in which the problems of nonexistent or insufficient health care, epidemic disease, and intractable suffering persist on the margins of engaging new cures. Despite medicine's triumphs over many forms of physical illness, ill-managed pain is still a part of even the more privileged lives.

THE NEW ANESTHESIA AND THE DEATH OF PAIN

From being one of the playthings of knowledge, it has been metamorphosed into one of its greatest triumphs; it has been, at one leap, transferred from the pages of toxicology to the latest, and almost the fairest, page of the healing art. ... next to the discovery of Franklin, it is the second and greatest contribution of the New World to science, and it is the first great addition to the medical art. (Wakely 1847)

By now it is a commonplace that on or about October 16, 1846, in Massachusetts General Hospital, Boston, a revolution took place not simply in how pain was treated, but, more fundamentally, in how it was imagined. The success of Surgeon John Collins Warren's use of anesthesia virtually overshadowed the failure of the surgery itself, an attempt to remove a tumor from the face of a young printer who had received dentist William Morton's "Letheon Gas." In England, as in America, doctors and patients hailed the victory over pain.

Pernick and others have documented the ways in which this was a patchy revolution: anesthesia use was based in part on a "calculus of [individual] suffering" that assumed each person had an essential sensitivity to pain based on embodied identities such as race, class, gender, and age. It is clear, however, that after 1846, many British doctors and patients looked at the prospect of surgery in completely new ways, having debated, reconsidered, and reconstituted the very concept of pain. Before, pain had been variously considered a necessary and important evil or an actual good: pain was a meaningful punishment of humankind's transgression against God or natural laws, a moral medicine and tonic, an informative vital sign, and a key facilitator of natural processes including childbirth and healing after surgery. (For an excellent summary of attitudes about pain both before and after 1846, see Pernick [1985], especially Chapters 3 and 4.)

Once surgical anesthesia was accepted as successful and morally valid, the debates about surgical and obstetric anesthesia allowed pain to be reformulated as an experience with limited redemptive value. Pain was not just a sign of disease but a pathological condition—even an "evil" in itself. After 1846, pain became a sensation that could be eradicated without disrupting either the theological or the natural order. And "anesthesia," which earlier had been a diagnosis, was now revalued as a "good" in the appropriate contexts, a facilitator or even an agent of cure, much as pain had originally been theorized (Christophers 1846).

Anesthesia had been an option for nonsurgical pain relief before 1846. Doctors used ether and chloroform as antispasmodics and to provide rest and a release from pain during chronic and terminal illnesses, particularly respiratory illnesses like phthisis (pulmonary tuberculosis). The success of surgical anesthesia stimulated and complemented research into new pain therapies for nonsurgical contexts, as well as putting a new spin on ether and chloroform. In terms of overall effects on attitudes toward pain relief, as well as on research for more effective pain treatments, both the debates about surgical anesthesia and the research generated by its success may well have helped to improve the treatment of nonsurgical pain.

Ironically, however, pain outside the realm of surgery is not a particularly visible subject to the researcher of this era. While pain and freedom from pain are often referenced in case narratives (probably with an additional emphasis on "free from pain" in post-1846 surgical cases), only selected works before the late 1880s make nonsurgical pain their focus. It is almost as if any kind of pain that is not related to surgery exists underground in medical texts after 1846; it is there but must be looked for in a very active way, more so because the *Index Medicus* does not track pain as a subject until the late 1880s. (For example, "neuralgia" is not indexed under "pain" in this period.)

It is in this context that I introduce provincial doctors William Dale and John Kent Spender, and London doctor Herbert Snow. All three achieved the M.D. degree; two were members of the Royal College of Physicians (Spender in England, Dale in Scotland), and Snow was a member of the less prestigious Royal College of Surgeons. All three published in the *Lancet*, *British Medical Journal*, and (significantly) *Practitioner*, and garnered other forms of peer respect (Peterson 1978; Bynum and Wilson 1992). (For a discussion of these "general professional periodicals" and their readership, see Bynum and Wilson [1992] and the other essays in Bynum et al. [1992]. For a discussion of the professionalization of doctors and the professional and social hierarchy in which physicians were superior to surgeons, see Peterson [1978].) At the same time, none of these doctors' writings on pain appears to have been central to mainstream medical discourse, and their ideas became less so as time went on.

WILLIAM DALE ADVOCATES OPIATES FOR DYING PATIENTS

William Dale was a surgeon and later, physician, whose essay on "The State of the Medical Profession in Great Britain and Ireland" won the Carmichael Prize of the Council of the Royal College of Surgeons, Ireland, in 1873 (Peterson 1978). The prize essay's concern both with established practitioners and with the education, including moral education, of medical students, suggests the similar dimension of his writing on pain. Dale remains something of a mystery. We know that he wrote on chorea and also on the management of consumption. He probably retired to Truro in Cornwall in 1900. "On Pain, and Some of the Remedies for its Relief" appeared in the *Lancet* from May to June, 1871. One of the first things we notice about Dale is that he was very literary, prone to allusions and attentive to language itself. The literary quality of his prose is partly indicative of the professionalization of medicine during the 19th century; many medical writers of this era produced corresponding textual evidence of their liberal arts education. Like many other writers of his time, for example, Dale is fond of Milton and draws on *Paradise Lost* to inaugurate his discussion:

> Pain is perfect misery, the worst
> Of evils; and, excessive, overturns
> All patience. (Dale 1871)

Significantly, this line is uttered to Satan by one of the rebel angels proposing to renew the attack on God with better weapons after they have lost the war in Heaven. The quotation, then, like other much-used literary references, takes on a new meaning in the specific context of pain discourse that it does not have in the plot of *Paradise Lost*; this changed meaning also suggests the degree to which literary references were used to establish the social authority of doctors, and implies that "literature" in the age of Matthew Arnold held claims to knowledge that are hard to establish today.

Dale alludes to Dickens and Burns as well, using these literary allusions to help him catalogue old and new pain remedies for then-fatal illnesses such as phthisis, asthma, heart disease, and cancer, and nonfatal painful conditions such as tetanus and neuralgia. Dale exemplifies how pain, while it can eradicate language in those who feel it, can also generate a proliferation of language and literariness in those who observe it. He writes, for example, that pain "is complained of as sharp, heavy, throbbing, stabbing, splitting, boring, burning, tearing, cutting, wearing." Dale is especially striking when he comments that words "are quite inadequate to describe" one scene of asthmatic suffering he has witnessed. It is "dreadful to remember the self-evident agony of this case, and difficult to contemplate without the deepest sympathy and pain, suffering which generally we can so inadequately relieve" (Dale 1871).

Pain gives Dale particular recourse to language and literariness in the context of his enthusiasm for pain medicine. He is an unconflicted advocate for using opiates, particularly to ease the process of dying:

> Opium is ... our chief medicine for relieving pain and procuring sleep—our right hand in practice. ... suffering humanity owes much to its virtues, and the physician could ill spare it in his battle with disease and pain. ... its effects are often wonderful, translating the poor patient from the state of the most intolerable torture to one of comparative ease and comfort—nay, entirely from Tartarus to Elysium. On the near approach of death, where much pain is endured, after having, as in duty bound, made the patient sensible of his condition, I see no reason why he may not be kept constantly under the influence of opium, or some other hypnotic, as a rule, so that, with the blessing of God, his misery and pain may be lessened or removed as he passes through the gloomy shades of death. (Dale 1871)

Like William Munk, who was more famous for publishing biographical data on the Royal College of Surgeons than for his still-used book on the care of the dying, *Euthanasia* (1887), Dale cites the work of Thomas Watson in *Principles and Practice of Physic* (1836), which discusses pain in the context of his larger comments on modes of dying (N. Hughes and D. Clark, unpublished manuscript).

While the pain of dying is a special case for doctors then and now, Dale's enthusiasm for opiates is not restricted to deathbed scenes, and his involvement in the language the patient uses to articulate pain is a reminder of strains in the art of medicine that do not necessarily die out with the advent of anesthesia and the silent, controlled patient. His one reference to the dangers of dependency is a moralizing footnote on reputed morphine use by women patients after they have been released from medical care:

> This remedy, like every good thing, is being abused. It is stated that some women, after having been hypodermically treated under medical surveillance, are in the habit of injecting morphia ... on their own responsibility, when suffering from slight neuralgic pains, mental depression, or severe ennui—just as the drunkard takes his dram. So easily are bad habits generated where the moral power is weak. (Dale 1871)

The comment also points to one important thread in the history of pain relief, discussed by Pernick (1985): the effect of gender on the assessment of suffering. Another theme, the dividing line between "real" and "hysterical" pain, was also an issue of debate during the 19th century. Dale's concern is

clearly with the moral failings of specific patients, not the fear of iatrogenically generated dependency, and no such fear attenuates his support of doctors' use of opiates for pain relief.

JOHN KENT SPENDER AFFIRMS THE DOCTOR'S
DUTY TO RELIEVE PAIN

The next writer, John Kent Spender, was a Bath practitioner, Surgeon to
the Eastern Dispensary and later Physician to the Mineral Water Hospital. In
these capacities, Spender attended to many patients who had come to this
fashionable watering-hole for a range of therapies for chronic illness. While
Spender's father had also been a physician, Spender himself was the head of
an intensely literary family; his wife was a prolific novelist and his son,
John Alfred (1862–1942), became a journalist and the editor of the *West-
minster Gazette*. Spender is credited with coining the term "osteoarthritis"
and also wrote about gout.

Spender's *Therapeutic Means for the Relief of Pain* (1874), like Dale's
essay, catalogues and comments on pharmacological and constitutional or
"moral" remedies for pain with reference to their effects on various illnesses, not all of them fatal, but all of them painful. He shares both Dale's
literariness and his tendency to rhapsodize about various medications, as
well as his concern for language itself, asserting:

> [We] depend upon the sufferer of pain for all information about its amount
> and its quality. A subtle essence has to be translated into words: the words
> themselves are used in different senses by different people: nor can we set
> up a standard by which the use of those words shall be governed. ... The
> enquirer himself may be unintelligent, or impatient, or perverse; and so bars
> may be interposed on his side to the discovery and reception of the truth.
> (Spender 1874)

Spender frames his ethos of pain relief in religious terms and seems to
speak directly to earlier debates surrounding surgical anesthesia. He characterizes the relief of pain as "not only a scientific duty, but a religious duty,"
asserting that "the duty of relieving Pain stands foremost with every truthful
physician; it is the grandest badge of his Art, and the best illustration of the
progress of the Economy of Medicine. ... a theme which is almost divine,
and which flows over with tender pity to weak and suffering Man" (Spender
1874).

As Spender constructs the doctor, he defines himself and his profession
on the basis of his ability to relieve pain. The point is not that Spender

emphasizes his own compassion, but rather that he continually returns to pain relief as a defining feature of his professional role, much as pre-anes-thesia surgeons like Robert Liston defined their merit by speed, itself a measure of compassion. Spender moderates between the desire to conquer pain and the refusal to see himself or his patients as failures if anesthesia does not always work:

> Writers on Neuralgia may disparage the inhalation of Chloroform because it does not give us that complete mastery over Pain which we rightfully crave. But it is good to do what we can, even if we cannot do all that we would. The practitioner who always carries a little store of Chloroform about him will joyfully discover many opportunities which he did not expect for his benevolent intervention. (Spender 1874)

Spender is explicitly critical of others in his profession who are reluc-tant to adopt the means available for patient care:

> No patients are more grateful for this discovery in therapeutic science, and none look forward with such piteous eagerness to the morning and evening visits of the doctor who brings the merciful boon. Seldom does it afford more pride and pleasure to be a physician! Certain is it that the medical man who (from ignorance or timidity) withholds hypodermic medicine from a patient afflicted with cancer, is guilty of indirectly permitting a huge quantity of unnecessary pain; and with our present knowledge ... he is totally without excuse. (Spender 1874)

This stance on pain relief extends to the dying, where "one of the chief blessings of Opium is to help us in granting the boon of a comparatively painless death. ... we may, without extinguishing consciousness, take away the sharp edge of suffering, and make the departure from this world less full of terror" (Spender 1874).

Finally, Spender speaks out against those professional emphases that overshadow the practice of compassionate care:

> Before we can relieve a given pain, says the philosopher, we must find out its cause. Wise and deep saying! Then if we fail to know the cause, is the pain to go on unhindered? ... If we see a man bleeding to death, must we refuse to stop the living tide until we know for certain where the blood comes from? (Spender 1887)

Spender advocates a particular balance of care and research, writing that:

> [T]he greatest hindrance to our successful treatment of neuralgia has been our obstinate theorizing about its etiology. While we are busy in classifying

our supposed *materies morbi* … and are applying our chemical and dynamical drugs accordingly, we are apt to forget the simple clinical fact that a human being lies in agony by our side, and supplicates relief for that one symptom: pain. Let us, if we can, first utterly overwhelm and abolish this pain; perhaps it will never return; but at all events, when our patient is in a grateful stupor, there will be time to philosophise about the origin of the malady. (Spender 1860)

Spender is emphatic about the issue of the physician as ethical man. As he writes, "A medical man himself may be a good and powerful anodyne, by reason of his truthfulness, self-sacrifice, and loyal care. Without the analgesic touch of sympathy all our cleverness is but dust and ashes" (Spender 1874). He also reminds his readers that doctors can be patients as well, a precursor, as in so much of his work, of current work in medical humanities. A final significant thread of Spender's work that will recur in Snow is the belief that pain itself is not only a sign of pathology, but has the power to "wear and destroy organic structures" (Spender 1887), an idea suggestive of John Liebeskind's argument that "Pain *Can* Kill."

HERBERT SNOW PROMOTES OPIATES FOR CANCER CURE

When he is remembered at all, Herbert Snow is remembered as the originator in 1896 of the medicament later known as the "Brompton cocktail" (also known as Brompton's cocktail, Brompton's mixture, or *mist euphorians*), which David Clark discusses in detail in Chapter 6. Snow was for 29 years a surgeon at the London Cancer Hospital, now the Royal Marsden Hospital, one of the few hospitals created in the Victorian era to house and care for cancer patients and others perceived as incurables. William Marsden founded the hospital in 1851 after seeing what his wife experienced as she died of cancer. Snow became senior surgeon at the Cancer Hospital before his resignation in 1906 at age 59. After he left the Marsden, he virtually disappeared from professional debates about cancer; he spent his final years deeply involved in the antivivisectionist movement (Royal Cancer Hospital 1951).

Snow's many works on cancer treatment include *On The Palliative Treatment of Incurable Cancer, with an Appendix on the Use of the Opium-Pipe* (1890), *The Path of Improvement in Cancer Treatment* (1893), and *Twenty-Two Years' Experience in the Treatment of Cancerous and Other Tumours* (1898). His stance on pain relief is uniquely proactive. "The practice of withholding opium until compelled by pain to resort to its use," he asserts, "merits unmeasured condemnation from every point of view," recommending instead that:

[T]he golden rule in cancer not amenable to cure by surgical eradication, is *to initiate at the earliest moment the administration of opium or morphia* in small, continued, gradually-increased doses. ... Making certain local exceptions, the patient with an incurable malignant tumour should thus become permanently subject to the morphine habit, purposely induced. (Snow 1893)

Not only his advocacy of intentionally and iatrogenically produced physical dependency, but also his focus on incurable cases, make Snow unusual among his peers. He departs from Dale and Spender in his more emphatic assertion of what they merely suggest—that certain analgesics not only can cloak (literally, palliate) pain, but also perform a genuinely therapeutic function by "checking the malignant cell-proliferation" (Snow 1890). "In the case of incurable cancerous patients," he writes, "the induction of an opium or morphia habit appears to be the most powerful and useful weapon we possess, not only for the relief of pain, but for the prolongation of life, and even for checking the development of the disease" (Snow 1890). The theoretical basis for this claim is that pain sensation itself causes cells to proliferate and also that pain is most intensely experienced in the cancers that have neurotic causes: "it is reasonable to anticipate that any drug tending to promote mental tranquillity should also check the progress of a disorder seemingly brought about by the absence of these conditions" (Snow 1890). Snow in his last publications is somewhat more conservative in his claims for opiates, and he advocates (as do the others) a proper balance in the practice of medicine; for him this balance means the integration of surgical and medical treatment. He stands by the belief, however, that pain relief in certain cases is not simply palliative, but also effective in arresting the growth of cancer.

Even more than Spender, Snow is explicitly critical of his profession and its ineffective practices of caring for cancer patients, suggesting that there is some basis for Morris's claim that the feeble and half-hearted treatment of pain was an accepted part of medical practice. Doctors are overly enamored of the latest and most exciting wave in medical methods, whereas:

Humanly speaking, the path of improvement which I have attempted imperfectly to indicate, would seem at present to lie far more in the better use of weapons long ready to our hand, than in the discovery of new. No one can pretend that the former have hitherto been employed in other than the most feeble and half-hearted fashion. (Snow 1893)

Further, Snow judges that his peers are ineffectual in their responses to pain, and thus encourage patients to use alternative medicines. "In the matter of medical treatment, the attitude of many orthodox practitioners towards cancer—'operate, or failing this, do nothing'—besides being commonly unwarranted by the facts, naturally urges resort to the quack" (Snow 1893).

Snow's disputes with his profession about the nature of cancer may have contributed to his disappearance from the map of the cultural history of pain relief. According to his somewhat brief obituary:

> [Snow was in his early career] a keen critic of the theories ... in vogue ... [and] later in his career he promulgated theories of cancer which in their turn were criticized, and the latter part of his life was largely given up in an attempt to demonstrate the futility of physiological research as a means of promoting medical science. From 1908 on he was consulting surgeon to the National Antivivisection Hospital at Battersea. (Anonymous 1930)

The last published evidence I can find of Snow's contributions to the clinical conversation about pain relief and cancer comes in a discussion of uterine cancer at the British Medical Association Meeting of 1905. Snow asserts: "I submit that no one who systematically treats inoperable cases medicinally with opium and cocaine will fail to recognize the merits of these drugs in arresting the disease, *or will invoke these egregious failures— x rays, radium, high-tension currents*" (Snow 1905; emphasis added).

Snow demonstrates the combined pressure to devise a cure for cancer and the desire not to be caught up in "egregious failures" whose ultimate damage is to the patient. At the same time, it is important to recognize Snow's differences from Spender and Dale. Partly because he practiced in a hospital devoted to the treatment of cancer, itself the site of increasing interest in methods of cure, Snow's advocacy of opiates attempted to reframe cancer itself from an incurable to a curable disease, and to position the tools of care as the agents of cure, a hypothesis the other doctors only imply. The same investment in the notion of cure is inherent in Snow's critique of his profession and of its ineffective practices in caring for cancer patients. More than any of the others, Snow demonstrates the real tension permeating cancer as it became, as had surgery since 1846, a subject in which thinking about cure rather than treatment alone transformed the universe of what could be thought not simply about pain, but also about the doctor's possible role in relation to it and his patient.

As we look beyond Snow, it becomes more difficult to locate the emphasis on care so clearly integral to the words of Dale and Spender. Few of the cancer hospitals founded in the 19th century survived to the 20th, and those hospitals that did survive had an increasing emphasis on research (Murphy 1989). But these writers all testify that there was a discourse on pain, care, and the art of medicine that did not disappear in the shadow of surgical pain relief or even in the wake of the drive toward scientific cures that followed the introduction of the germ theory. This persistent discourse should remind us to always balance our attention to larger trends in the epistemology of medicine with local analysis of medical practice, to look outside what is indexed, and to consider not just how pain is defined and theorized, but also how patient care is practiced and narrated around the pervasive issue of pain.

ACKNOWLEDGMENTS

Research for this chapter was supported by grants from the National Endowment for the Humanities and the California State University–San Marcos University Senate and College of Arts and Sciences Faculty Development Committee. The participants in the Second Annual History of Pain Symposium at UCLA offered enthusiastic suggestions on an early draft; the outside reader for this volume contributed invaluable revision advice at a later stage. I am hugely indebted to Marcia Meldrum for her gracious help with successive versions of the chapter; for her encouragement, patience, and generosity; and for her remarkable ability to bring together a diverse group of academics and professionals and inspire them to coalesce into an interdisciplinary community.

REFERENCES

Anonymous. Important American discovery. *London Lancet* 1847:156.
Anonymous. Epitome of current medical literature: sleeplessness in children. *BMJ* 1906; 10:1298.
Anonymous. Herbert Snow, M.D. Lond. Obituary. *Lancet* 1930; (Nov):1212–1213.
Bynum WF, Wilson JC. Periodical knowledge: medical journals and their editors in nineteenth-century Britain. In: Bynum WF, Lock S, Porter R (Eds). *Medical Journals and Medical Knowledge*. London: Routledge, 1992, pp 29–48.
Bynum WF, Lock S, Porter R (Eds). *Medical Journals and Medical Knowledge*. London: Routledge, 1992.
Christophers JC. Anaesthesia, treated by electro-magnetism, with observation on injury from the injudicious use of the cold hip-bath. *London Lancet* 1846; 326–327.
Dale W. On pain, and some of the remedies for its relief. *Lancet* 1871; (13 May):641–642; (20 May):679–680; (3 June):739–741; (17 June):816–817.
Davus M. Objects to be gained through the artificial induction of trance. *Blackwood's Edinburgh Magazine* 1847; 62:166–177.
Foucault M. *The Birth of the Clinic: An Archeology of Medical Perception*. New York: Vintage, 1973.
Morris D. *The Culture of Pain*. Berkeley: University of California Press, 1991.
Morris D. An invisible history. *Clin J Pain* 1998; 14:191–196.

Munk W. *Euthanasia: Or, Medical Treatment in Aid of an Easy Death.* London: Longmans, Green, 1887.

Murphy CCS. From Friedenheim to hospice: a century of cancer hospitals. In: Granshaw L, Porter R (Eds). *The Hospital in History.* London: Routledge, 1989, pp 221–241.

Pernick M. *A Calculus of Suffering: Pain, Professionalism, and Anesthesia in Nineteenth-Century America.* New York: Columbia University Press, 1985.

Peterson MJ. *The Medical Profession in Mid-Victorian England.* Berkeley: University of California Press, 1978.

Rey R. *The History of Pain.* Wallace LE, Cadden JA, Cadden SW (Transl). Cambridge, MA: Harvard University Press, 1998.

Royal Cancer Hospital. *The Royal Cancer Hospital, Fulham Road, London, 1851–1951: A Short History of the Royal Cancer Hospital Prepared for the Centenary.* London: J.B. Shears, 1951.

Scarry E. *The Body in Pain: The Making and Unmaking of the World.* New York: Oxford University Press, 1985.

Smith A. *The Theory of Moral Sentiments.* London: George Bell, 1907.

Snow HL. *On the Palliative Treatment of Incurable Cancer: With an Appendix on the Use of the Opium-Pipe.* London: Churchill, 1890.

Snow HL. *The Path of Improvement in Cancer Treatment.* London: Morton and Burt, 1893.

Snow HL. Opium and cocaine in the treatment of cancerous disease. *BMJ* 1896; 2:718–719.

Snow HL. *Twenty-Two Years' Experience in the Treatment of Cancerous and Other Tumours.* London: Baillière, Tindall, and Cox, 1898.

Snow HL. Discussion of the diagnosis and treatment of cancer of the uterus. Seventy-Third Annual Meeting of the British Medical Association. *BMJ* 1905; Sept:702–703.

Spender JK. The hypodermic action of morphia. *BMJ* 1860; June:436–437.

Spender JK. *Therapeutic Means for the Relief of Pain.* London: Macmillan, 1874.

Spender JK. Remarks on 'analgesics.' *BMJ* 1887; April:819–822.

Stanley P. *For Fear of Pain: British Surgery, 1790–1850.* Amsterdam: Editions Rodopi, 2003.

Wakely T. Editorial. *London Lancet,* 1847; 1:241.

Correspondence to: Martha Stoddard Holmes, PhD, Department of Literature and Writing Studies, 6th Floor, Craven Hall, 333 Twin Oaks Boulevard, California State University, San Marcos, CA 92096-0001, USA. Email: mstoddar@csusm.edu.

Opioids and Pain Relief: A Historical Perspective,
Progress in Pain Research and Management, Vol.
25, edited by Marcia L. Meldrum, IASP Press,
Seattle, © 2003.

4

Take as Directed: The Dilemmas of Regulating Addictive Analgesics and Other Psychoactive Drugs

Caroline Jean Acker

*Department of History, Carnegie Mellon University,
Pittsburgh, Pennsylvania, USA*

Those seeking to restrict the use of opioids to authorized medical use have attempted to divide good drugs from bad drugs, good people from bad people, and good forms of use from bad forms of use. As this inconsistency suggests, the line separating legitimate medical use of drugs from use that is manifestly harmful to users, their immediate social networks, and society at large is not always easy to discern, let alone maintain. In a discussion of the social context of the prescribing and taking of medicines, Morgan (1983) wrote: "A cultural traffic in chemicals has always both served and been influenced by magical, mythological, and psychological forces."

This chapter provides a historical context for understanding the cultural traffic of chemicals (opioids and other psychoactive substances) across the shifting and complex boundary separating medical from nonmedical drug use in the United States. The idea of drug diversion from medical to non-medical use presupposes the existence of a line to be crossed, a chasm that separates legitimate patients from street users. This divide has not always existed; it is a product of the intertwined moves in the Progressive Era to eliminate forms of drug use considered "vicious" (related to vice) and to consolidate medical authority around scientific medicine.

MEDICAL REFORMS AND PATIENTS' EXPECTATIONS

By the late 19th century, the prevalence of domestic medicine that charac-terized the Jacksonian era was being challenged in various ways. Increasingly, patients were seeking care in hospitals rather than at home. The bacteriological revolution, which would help transform both medical and popular ideas about disease, was under way, and the expanding print media gave it lots of coverage (Tomes 1998). The meaning of "medicine" was also undergoing change. From the 1870s, the American Medical Association (AMA) had been subjecting medicines to chemical analysis and undermining the groundless or exaggerated claims that sellers made for various remedies (American Medical Association 1911, 1921, 1936). But for many, taking care of their own health and treating disease themselves or within the family and the home remained important.

Medicines had long been taken to relieve symptoms, and their workings were explained in a humoral framework that interpreted symptoms in a medical system that lay persons could understand (Rosenberg 1979). These symptoms included fever, sweating, diarrhea, coughing, and pain. A medicine that made one feel better was a good medicine by definition, and patients knew which medicines had improved their sense of comfort or well-being. Opium and, later, morphine were powerful relievers of diarrhea, coughing, and pain. Even when they were not sick, people drank tonics to lift their spirits and maintain health. In this holistic framework, medicines and pick-me-ups were not always sharply demarcated, and a host of purveyors offered products to meet the demand for home-based health care and health maintenance.

In the Progressive Era, the related drives to reduce or eliminate alcohol consumption, reform the medical profession, and reduce contamination and chicanery in the marketing of food and drugs contributed to the creation of the "soft drink." Products like Coca Cola, whose original formulation contained cocaine, were changed from tonics promoted to improve health and functioning to beverages drunk simply to slake thirst, taste good, and offer that mildest of therapeutic benefits, refreshment.

In the same period, reformers transformed the institutions of medicine, and the ethical pharmaceutical industry linked its interests to those of the reforming physicians. This transformation influenced how patients thought about disease, therapeutics, and medicines. A functional view of the body as a system and disease as a derangement of that system's physiology was gradually replaced by an ontological view of diseases as having an independent existence. The 18th-century idea that fevers could mutate from one disease to another in the body of a unique patient gave way to a concept of distinct and specific diseases. Systemic pathology, in which disease was understood as affecting the whole body, was replaced by localized pathology, in which disease was understood as acting at a specific tissue or cell site.

Therapeutic ideas shifted from a holistic to a reductionist view, from an emphasis on the individual as unique to an emphasis on disease as uniform in all cases. In practice, this view meant a shift from shaping treatment differently for every case to prescribing a similar treatment for all cases of the same disease.

For physicians and patients, a praiseworthy medicine had long been "good for what ails you," one that affected the whole system and relieved a broad range of symptoms. As diseases were reframed in terms of localized pathology, pharmacologists sought medicines that targeted one or a few specific indications, acting at a local site in the body and attacking the cause of disease rather than treating the symptoms.

Scientific pharmacology developed new theories of medical efficacy and new methods in the search for improved medicines. The isolation of active compounds from traditional plant medicines (such as the derivation of morphine from opium) and the theory that molecular structure determined pharmacological action led to a profusion of novel naturally occurring, semi-synthetic, and synthetic compounds to be tested for pharmacological action. Traditional medicine often consisted of combinations of ingredients hawked as secret and uniquely efficacious formulas, but the products of the new pharmacology consisted of single compounds. The scientific norm of publishing results undermined the desirability of mystification in advertising a superior medicine. Pharmaceutical companies joining the scientific bandwagon shunned the advertising methods of nostrum hucksters in favor of advertising only to physicians. They relied on patents to protect the market share for their products, while the university-based scientists with whom they collaborated published the drug's synthesis and actions in the scientific literature.

This process of transformation was not always smooth or neat, as illustrated by a Maxfield Parrish poster advertising No-To-Bac. The makers of No-To-Bac claimed that their multi-ingredient secret formula could cure the tobacco habit, an affliction only recently described by Progressive reformers in their debate over whether drug habits constituted diseases or vices. Parrish's visually powerful illustration, depicting No-To-Bac as a knight slaying a dragon, exemplified the rise of a technologically and psychologically sophisticated advertising industry that drug manufacturers have used ever since.

When traditional medicine was transformed into scientific biomedicine, it lost some of what was important to patients—holism and the personal or spiritual meaning of illness (Kleinman 1988). Patients' nostalgia for these lost qualities has shaped their negotiations with physicians and their responses to psychoactive medications. In the late 20th century, patients hungered both for the miracles promised by scientific medicine and for the sense of meaning conferred by more traditional forms of care.

MEDICAL AND NONMEDICAL USE OF OPIATES

Opioids have always been central in the tensions between medical and nonmedical use. Morphine emerged in 1805 as the first medicine to be isolated as a pure compound from a plant source, and in the 1850s it became the first medication to be injected hypodermically, for the treatment of facial neuralgia (Howard-Jones 1947).

A well-known pattern of morphine use in the late 19th century was typified by middle-aged, middle-class women taking morphine provided by their physicians for a variety of discomforts (Courtwright 1982). This pattern exemplifies the shift from self-medication to medication use dependent on a physician's authorization. For decades, women had taken opium and, later, morphine, for menstrual pain, and many women began taking opioids this way. As young women went through menarche, their mothers taught them to take opium or morphine to relieve menstrual cramps (Acker, in press). However they were introduced to the drug, some women found that it assuaged a range of psychological discomforts, including stresses related to their class and gender roles. In a social world where women were stigmatized if they drank or smoked, a physician's prescription provided a socially legitimate way to manage feelings by consuming a psychoactive drug. Physicians, in turn, operated in a competitive, overcrowded profession, and many were loathe to turn down requests for medicine from a class of patients well able to pay fees, to speak well or ill of their physician to friends, and to influence the decisions other family members would make about where to seek care. The availability of the hypodermic syringe enabled subcutaneous injection, a more powerful route of administration than swallowing the drug, and one more likely to lead to addiction. This pattern formed part of a more general trend of growing medical authority and the medicalization of wide-ranging behavioral issues.

In the 1890s, some physicians, especially those interested in the larger reform of the profession, sounded the alarm over the prevalence of iatrogenic addiction resulting from such prescribing practices. Reducing the prescribing of opioids became an important plank in the reform platform (Acker 1995b). Rhetorically, the pitiful image of the morphine-addicted woman like Mary Tyrone in Eugene O'Neill's *A Long Day's Journey into Night* was useful in motivating reform and portraying reformers as exercising enlightened compassion consistent with the emerging scientific medicine.

Soon after Bayer introduced heroin as a cough remedy in 1898, young men in working-class neighborhoods in America's cities discovered that the drug provided powerful euphoric and calmative effects and began sharing it in poolrooms and dance halls (Courtwright 1982; Acker 2001). At least by

1910, some had discovered that by crushing the heroin tablets and sniffing the powder, they could achieve a more intense euphoria than when they swallowed the pill. This pattern of use fell squarely within the spatial, cultural, and behavioral zone of vice that Progressive Era reformers sought to eradicate; over the ensuing decades, heroin addiction would come to symbolize the most depraved and stubborn form of nonmedical drug use. But, as clinical records from the 1920s show, when these early addicts sought treatment, they reported many of the same motives for use as did the middle-class women who used morphine in the late 19th century and as do heroin addicts presenting for treatment in addiction programs today: "It makes me feel normal," or "Sometimes a gloomy day would get me started using again" (Acker 2001).

THE SEARCH FOR A NONADDICTIVE ANALGESIC

The Harrison Narcotic Act, passed in 1914, banned the use of opiates, cocaine, and a few other drugs except as administered or authorized by a physician. The commitment to prohibition of disapproved drug use implied a natural division of drugs into distinct categories of safe or dangerous, useful or vicious. But drugs like morphine, which remained essential in medical practice but were also used in ways we would now call recreational, posed ongoing problems. The language of Harrison confined the legal use of opiates to that authorized by physicians in the course of proper professional practice. The Supreme Court essentially withheld ambulatory treatment from addicts by its 1919 interpretation of the narcotic act as forbidding the prescribing of opiates in addiction treatment. Physicians, pharmaceutical manufacturers, and policy makers have ever since faced the dilemma of devising best medical practice for improving therapeutics with these highly useful, but addictive compounds (Musto 1973).

Their dilemma formed the context for launching a decades-long (and still ongoing) search for a nonaddicting analgesic that would be as effective a pain reliever as morphine (Acker 1997). Rice (this volume) describes this quest in terms of opioid chemistry and pharmacology. I will discuss the chemical, pharmacological, and clinical research toward the goal of a nonaddicting analgesic that was coordinated and overseen by the National Research Council (NRC). In 1929, the NRC took over the functions of the Committee on Drug Addictions created by the Bureau of Social Hygiene, a result of Rockefeller philanthropy whose main focus was the problem of prostitution. Later renamed the Committee on Drug Addiction and Narcotics, the group now functions as the College on Problems of Drug Dependence.

While still under Rockefeller auspices, the committee became an active participant in the League of Nations' Opium Advisory Committee, which sought to determine the legitimate needs of countries like the United States that depended on opiate importation for medical use, and to regulate the world's supply and distribution (McAllister 2000). In the late 1920s, committee head Lawrence Dunham conceived an idea for identifying the leakage points through which opiates passed from the legitimate medical trade to the illicit market. At that time, the processing of opium into morphine or heroin occurred almost entirely in pharmaceutical plants in Europe; diversion to the illicit market occurred either directly from some of these plants or after the processed drugs had entered the wholesale market.

Dunham proposed tagging batches of morphine or heroin with a compound that would be nontoxic when consumed by the patient or street user, but would turn a characteristic color with the addition of a reagent, thus enabling authorities to trace diverted supplies to the factories where they had been produced. Despite some promising chemical candidates, safety concerns prevented this project from being carried out (Acker 2001). By contrast, the heroin entering the illicit market today is typically produced in the countries where the opium poppies are grown, and its trafficking and marketing channels are entirely separate from those for licit drugs authorized for medical use.

Dunham recognized that the bacteriological revolution was being succeeded by a pharmacological revolution, in which an ever-increasing stream of new compounds would be devised and tested for medical usefulness. Just as heroin had resulted from pharmaceutical research, so, too, would other new compounds possessing serious liabilities, including a seductive attraction for people seeking to alter their consciousness and the potential to cause addiction (Acker 2001).

Along with central nervous system (CNS) depressants like opiates, pharmaceutical stimulants were subject to diversion. Amphetamine was introduced as a decongestant in the 1930s; its capacity to sustain physical and mental endurance over long periods quickly attracted users seeking to boost their energy. The Benzedrine inhaler was first marketed in 1932. The American writer William Burroughs used the inhalers for their stimulant effect; crime fiction author James Ellroy encountered them as a child. By 1946, amphetamines had 39 indications. Students, bohemians, truck drivers, and airplane pilots all took advantage of their stimulant properties. Other marketers offered their own amphetamine products when the Smith Kline and French patent expired in 1949. Up to half of the amphetamines produced were diverted to the illicit market.

Smith Kline and French added denatured picric acid to Benzedrine inhalers to discourage people from eating the wicks; users ate them anyway. Courtwright (2001) claims that Smith Kline and French promoted amphetamine "so aggressively for so many conditions that leakage was bound to occur." For example, the company recommended dextroamphetamine, marketed as Dexedrine, for diet control. In a process Courtwright calls drug democratization, heavy advertising by manufacturers and heavy prescribing by physicians help set the stage for illegitimate or excessive use. These abuses trigger a regulatory or legal response, often prohibition, which in turn is typically followed by illicit manufacture (Courtwright 2001).

The search for the nonaddicting analgesic, conceived in a period when diversion from legal opiate manufacture was the main source of illicit addictive drugs, has continued to the present, long after illicit production has become standard practice. By developing an analgesic that neither produced euphoria nor induced addiction, the project's originators hoped to end the need to track morphine supplies and to forestall their diversion to the illicit market.

The Committee on Drug Addiction researchers began their work in 1929. Under the leadership of Lyndon Small at the University of Virginia, chemists working on the quest for the nonaddicting analgesic produced hundreds of compounds over the course of the 1930s. The compounds were tested in animals at the University of Michigan in the laboratory of pharmacologist Nathan Eddy. Those deemed promising were sent for clinical testing to the Addiction Research Laboratory at the U.S. Public Health Service Narcotic Hospital in Lexington, Kentucky.

One of these compounds, Metopon, illustrates both the kind of progress made from the 1930s through the 1950s and the attendant problems of regulation. Metopon represented what Rice (this volume) has called the "proof of principle," vindication of the idea that the analgesic property of morphine could be uncoupled from its addictiveness. In preparing to test new compounds in humans to determine their addictiveness, Public Health Service physician Clifton Himmelsbach had developed a quantitative means of measuring the severity of the withdrawal syndrome, the pattern of runny nose, muscle twitches, nausea, vomiting, diarrhea, and other symptoms that follow abrupt cessation of opioid administration in an addicted person. This method enabled him to graph the timing and severity of onset of specific symptoms. Then, working from the hypothesis that any drug that quickly and reliably relieved these withdrawal symptoms was itself addicting in the same manner as morphine, he established an addictiveness assay: he would stabilize opioid addicts on doses of morphine that kept them comfortable;

then he would substitute a test drug for the morphine, and watch. If the subject developed withdrawal symptoms, then the test drug was presumed to be nonaddicting. However, if the subject remained comfortable and no symptoms of withdrawal ensued, the drug's capacity to stave off withdrawal was prima facie evidence of its addictiveness.

Metopon was addictive, although not as powerfully so as morphine. Himmelsbach's graph showing how Metopon performed in his morphine-substitution addictiveness assay indicated that addicts did manifest some mild signs of withdrawal when they were switched from morphine to Metopon, and that, when Metopon administration was stopped, the subjects experienced more severe signs of withdrawal, although not as severe as those associated with morphine. Nevertheless, Metopon's combination of analgesic potency with reduced addiction liability helped persuade the Public Health Service to take over support for the research when the Rockefeller Foundation withdrew the funding that had carried the project through the mid-1930s. The Addiction Research Center at Lexington became the accepted site for testing new compounds for addictive potential, and pharmaceutical companies from around the world sent compounds there for testing if they suspected that they might be addictive (Acker 1995a).

Chemist Lyndon Small and pharmacologist Nathan Eddy moved to the National Institute of Health (then still a single institute) in 1939; there, they and their laboratory groups could maintain closer coordination than had been possible between Charlottesville and Ann Arbor. A growing number of new compounds—some derived from the morphine molecule and others produced synthetically—produced a range of effects that, in turn, suggested new chemical strategies. By the late 1940s, compounds could be classified based on whether they acted as agonists (producing morphine-like effects), or as antagonists (reversing the effects of morphine or similar drugs in the body).

NOVEL DRUGS PROVE SUSCEPTIBLE TO ABUSE

In the early 1950s at Small's laboratory at the National Institutes of Health, chemist Everette May began producing a set of new compounds based on the benzomorphan molecule that combined agonist and antagonist properties. Sydney Archer and his colleagues at the Sterling-Winthrop Research Institute built on May's work in 1964 to develop pentazocine, a mixed agonist-antagonist. The drug produced analgesia, and was apparently negligible in addictiveness as demonstrated by the Himmelsbach Abstinence Scale. When marketed as a prescription-only analgesic with the brand name

Talwin, it was not classed among the drugs requiring regulation under the Harrison Narcotic Act (Eddy 1973; Acker 1997).

Nevertheless, by the mid-1970s, pentazocine had aroused concern as a drug susceptible to abuse. Addicts typically have a preferred form of opioid, with heroin as the most common preference, both for pharmacological reasons and because of its ready availability through the efficient illicit market. But when the preferred opioid is hard to find, addicts will resort to others they can more easily obtain. Desperate junkies had presumably resorted to pentazocine to stave off withdrawal when heroin was in short supply. At some point, such an addict injected pentazocine shortly before or after taking the antihistamine pyribenzamine, probably for relief of allergy symptoms. To his surprise, the drugs worked synergistically to produce a euphoria similar to that produced by heroin. As word of this unexpected effect traveled through social networks of heroin users, the diversion of pentazocine rose to levels that drew the attention of regulators.

Harris Isbell at the Addiction Research Center had hypothesized in the early 1950s that adding a small amount of an opioid antagonist to medications that had agonist effects would prevent these drugs from causing addiction in users (Eddy 1973). In 1983, Winthrop adopted this tactic to combat abuse of its pentazocine preparations by adding naloxone, a pure antagonist, to the drugs (Meier 2001a).

However, the adaptation of pentazocine to the drug-seeking behaviors of addicts exposed the inadequacy of the standard addictiveness assay, which had formed the basis for regulatory classification of drugs as addicting or nonaddicting. The assay could not determine the likelihood that a medication would be sought by addicts and thus enter the netherworld of street drugs. Moreover, the existing law that sought to divide drugs into two stark categories, addictive or nonaddictive, failed to reflect the chemical complexity created by the profusion of new opioid compounds with their range of agonist, antagonist, and mixed agonist-antagonist effects (Eddy 1973).

By the late 1950s, the NRC Committee on Drug Addiction and Narcotics recognized that the law's dichotomous classification system was too restrictive. The committee urged a series of schedules that would rank drugs in several categories representing various ratios of addiction liability to therapeutic value (Eddy 1973). Committee leaders still saw addicts as sociopaths who would not respond to ambulatory or maintenance treatment, but required long-term institutionalization. Their advocacy of more flexibility in medical use of analgesics ran ahead of their willingness to accept new ideas in the treatment of addiction, as evidenced by their disapproval of the idea of using methadone as a maintenance drug.

Wholesale diversion remained a serious problem under the legal regime then in place. Up to half of barbiturates and amphetamines were being diverted to the illicit market. The 1970 Controlled Substances Act put into law the scheduling plan urged by the Committee on Drug Addiction and Narcotics, creating the five schedules that remain in force to this day (Eddy 1973). Schedule I includes drugs with high addiction liability that are deemed to have no medical usefulness (the approval of heroin for medical use in some other countries and recent initiatives to explore the medical usefulness of marijuana remind us that a drug's supposed lack of medical usefulness is a contingent category). Schedules II through V include drugs with recognized medical uses and some degree of addiction liability; these schedules rank drugs in descending order of addictive potential.

The law also imposed manufacturing quotas that sharply reduced the volume of drugs manufactured in pharmaceutical plants and then diverted in large quantities to the illicit market. These quotas made it harder for drug dealers to carry out the levels of wholesale diversion that had prevailed through the 1950s and 1960s (Anthony 1983). In the 1970s, illicit marketers shifted to bootlegging and ingredient substitution. They took advantage of the product recognition achieved by pharmaceutical companies by making tablets or capsules that closely resembled known psychoactive drugs. These might contain varying amounts and combinations of the medicinal compound, another compound with similar effects, or inactive fillers.

For example, by the late 1970s, a profusion of black and yellow capsules bearing different numbers were being marketed as "speed." These typically contained combinations of over-the-counter stimulants, such as caffeine, ephedrine, and phenylpropanolamine, but they did not contain amphetamines, as users were led to believe by the capsules' superficial similarity to the prescription drugs. It took little capital investment to buy empty capsules marked to order and fill them with cheap, unregulated drugs (Pawlak 1980). By about 1980, grass roots drug information hotlines were overwhelmed by callers describing such capsules and asking about ingredients and risks (Passe 1981). Only when users sent capsules to street drug analysis laboratories, run by grass roots organizations and licensed by the Drug Enforcement Administration (DEA), did they learn of the deception. This episode, and the poisoning of Tylenol capsules in the same period, prompted manufacturers to stop using easily opened capsules for powdered medications.

Depressants attracted copycat entrepreneurs as well. Methaqualone, a CNS depressant that produces an alcohol-like intoxication, was widely sold in bootlegged tablets bearing the incised marking "Rorer 714" or "Lemmon 714" to mimic the appearance of the prescription drug best known by the trade name Quaalude. These tablets might well contain the advertised ingredient, but often they contained diazepam (Valium) rather than methaqualone.

Early in 1980, callers flooded drug hotlines with reports of alarming symptoms after taking imitation Quaaludes. Four symptom patterns emerged from the descriptions: immediate, powerful nausea and vomiting with headache; 24 hours or more of sleep and mental cloudiness; explosions of uncharacteristically angry or violent behavior; and toxic psychosis and suicidal impulses.

The first suspected culprit was phencyclidine, or PCP, also a popular street drug and the object of lurid portrayal in that year's media frenzy (Morgan and Kagan 1982). Stories about raving, violent behavior triggered by PCP lent credence to the hypothesis that this drug explained the rash of reports. However, samples sent to analysis laboratories failed to reveal PCP as an ingredient. The solution came when Up Front Drug Information, a grass roots organization in Miami founded in 1973, asked users to send in pills from batches linked to the bad reactions. Up Front's DEA-licensed pharmacologist, who managed its street-drug analysis laboratory, examined the pills. His quantitative analysis found that a single pill contained anywhere between 250 and 350 mg of diazepam—that is, 25 times a typical clinical dose or more. Others had stopped at qualitative analysis, and when diazepam, a common ingredient of the fake Quaaludes, turned up, they assumed they had analyzed uncontaminated tablets.

The symptoms that users had reported are all textbook symptoms of diazepam overdose. It is fortunate that diazepam has a such a broad margin of safety and that no one who had taken these pills had also consumed enough alcohol or other CNS depressants to create a lethal synergistic effect. Deaths from diazepam overdose, when it is taken alone, are virtually unheard of, and no deaths were attributed to these pills (Gellman and Ciancutti 1980).

In 2000 a new diversion story recalled some old themes. OxyContin, Purdue Pharma's time-released formulation of oxycodone introduced in 1995, was implicated in a pattern of diversion that contributed to an alarming increase in fatal opioid overdoses in many parts of the United States (Tough 2001). A time-released opioid analgesic has clear therapeutic utility: it achieves a stability of dose over 24 hours that relieves pain effectively without the fluctuations in relief, or side effects, associated with taking four to six pills at scheduled intervals. In a sense, a time-released tablet achieves the same result as the more arduous and chancy search for a compound with a longer duration of action; thus, OxyContin possesses advantages analogous to those of methadone over morphine or heroin in the treatment of opioid dependence. The product filled an emerging market niche. With the growth of the pain management field, a new generation of pain specialists and a vocal patient constituency had redefined the undertreatment of chronic pain as a major problem and the potential addiction of pain patients as a minor risk. These new attitudes legitimized more liberal prescribing of opioids for pain relief.

Street users, like the heroin sniffers of the early 1900s, quickly discovered that crushing the OxyContin tablet produced a potent sniffable powder. Crushing defeated the time-release mechanism so that a dose intended to enter the system gradually was delivered within minutes to the brain. In a characteristic narrative paradox, the media portrayed this phenomenon as both unprecedented and familiar, a uniquely horrifying case of a powerful drug wreaking havoc in American communities—just as many other drugs had done in the past.

News coverage showed parking lots jammed with vehicles as street users sought prescriptions from physicians who wrote wholesale prescriptions with little pretense of a physical examination (Meier 2001b). Reporters also described a pattern in which the rural elderly poor used their Medicare and Medicaid coverage to acquire OxyContin and then sold the pills on the street, for as much as $50 per tablet, to supplement their meager Social Security income. Early in 2002, media coverage reached a climax when prosecutors charged physicians with manslaughter and murder following the deaths of patients from overdoses of prescription OxyContin. In February, a Florida physician was convicted of manslaughter and sentenced to 63 years in prison for having prescribed OxyContin to four patients who died after taking the drug (Meier 2002a,b).

OxyContin was not the first time-released opioid analgesic to be put on the market; the product was modeled after MS Contin, a time-released form of morphine first marketed in Britain by a company that Purdue had acquired. According to Purdue, no notable problems arose with the earlier medication, either when given in hospitals or prescribed to outpatients. Why, then, did OxyContin become implicated in this rash of abuse?

Part of the answer lies in the prescribing patterns of physicians. As a time-released form of the drug contained in the combination of oxycodone and aspirin marketed as Percodan, OxyContin must have seemed to many physicians as suitable for moderate pain in cases where they were reluctant to prescribe morphine. Purdue specifically marketed OxyContin as a solution for the patient with persistent moderate pain for whom the standard drugs had not worked. The company provided physicians with tables showing equivalent doses of various analgesics to the recommended dose of OxyContin so that physicians could select the appropriate dose for a particular patient's pain. Many physicians undoubtedly welcomed a new option for dealing with the frustrating patient who repeatedly complained of unrelieved pain. And, as word spread of the drug's desirability—whether as an effective and easy-to-take analgesic or as a euphoriant that would stave off withdrawal symptoms from other narcotics—more patients began requesting the drug from physicians.

On the street user side, OxyContin abuse occurred in the context of the increase in heroin use in the mid-to-late 1990s, as the crack cocaine wave diminished. More specifically, OxyContin became problematic in many rural areas and small towns, which have less access to the illicit market in imported drugs than do the larger American cities (Tough 2001). Stimulants such as methamphetamine, produced in crude amateur laboratories in many rural locations in the United States, are used more commonly than opioids in these settings. To young rural drug users, OxyContin represented a relatively unfamiliar class of drug suddenly available in the form of a single crushable tablet that yielded a powerfully high dose.

This pattern displays characteristics typical of drug epidemics, from the gin scare in England in the 18th century to the crack epidemic of the 1980s. The common ingredients of such an episode are the introduction of a new psychoactive drug, or a new and more powerful form of a drug, into a new social context; the absence of social experience with the drug that would give rise to social norms encouraging moderation and curbing excess; and the presence of social turmoil or chronic socioeconomic disadvantage in the population to which the drug is introduced (Zinberg 1984). OxyContin was a powerful and comparatively unfamiliar drug whose advent in regions of rural poverty interacted with prevailing life patterns of managing that poverty and the accompanying medical indigence.

Those who took the drug to experience effects other than simple analgesia discovered its potency as a euphorigenic and calmative. Because they began use with a fairly high dose, they soon developed tolerance and moved rapidly toward dependence; a continuing market for prescriptions developed. The new cohort of opioid users had little access to the counsel of seasoned addicts. As habits reached high dose levels in a comparatively short time, sniffers shifted to injections, and inexperience with dose management and lack of knowledge about drug combinations contributed to sometimes lethal overdoses.

As the problem came to the attention of law enforcement officials and regulatory bodies, a new set of interests came into play. Prosecutors brought physicians to trial not just on the charge of improper prescribing, but on the higher-profile charges of manslaughter and murder when patients had died. Defense attorneys argued that their clients were simply conforming to new pain treatment norms. This argument effectively pitted the interests of pain patients against those of addicts. The two classes of patients face related problems of credibility in the doctor's office. Chronic pain patients must persuade physicians of the reality of their pain, which typically has no objective physiological correlate; in the United States, physicians have been conditioned by decades of AMA and DEA surveillance and sanctions to suspect that such patients may be addicts lying to try to obtain opioids (Acker 1995b). Many opioid addicts have feigned pain in just such an attempt and thus have earned physicians' distrust. Addicts have perhaps the greater problem of credibility in the doctor's office, to the extent that this same tradition has made physicians reluctant to accept them as patients, whether for their addiction or for other conditions they might suffer.

Hospital policy regarding addicted patients varies. At one hospital in Pittsburgh, Pennsylvania, attending physicians use their discretion in managing heroin addicts admitted for conditions related to drug use, such as systemic infections arising from abscesses at injection sites or for unrelated illness. Some physicians put these patients on methadone maintenance while they are in the hospital; others simply provide a palliative regimen, such as combinations of clonidine and benzodiazepines, to ease the withdrawal symptoms inevitable in the absence of the addictive drug. At another Pittsburgh hospital, heroin-addicted patients receive methadone while their medical condition is stabilized; when hospital staff determine it is medically safe, patients are switched to palliative medications. Under such a regimen, patients sometimes check out of the hospital against medical advice as soon as they feel able to do so (personal communications, anonymous participants of Prevention Point Pittsburgh needle exchange program, 1999–2002).

The almost concurrent rise of chronic pain management and addiction medicine as new specialties, both faced with the need to establish credibility and legitimacy, has also affected the context in which OxyContin was diverted and abused. As noted, defense attorneys argued that their physician clients were following new, enlightened practice in prescribing opioids liberally to legitimate chronic pain patients. This defense ploy pitted the two specialties against each other.

In 2001 the College on Problems of Drug Dependence responded to the media attention to opioid diversion by appointing a task force to examine the issue. The college, present-day successor to the Committee on Drug Addiction and thus long involved in the assessment of drugs' abuse liability, has the mission of providing a scientific basis to guide drug policy. The task force's report reviewed evidence indicating a rise in prevalence of nonmedical use of opioid analgesics, primarily hydrocodone and oxycodone. For example, comparing Drug Abuse Warning Network reports of the number of times specific drugs were linked to users' emergency room visits with the number of prescriptions written for various opioids, the report authors noted a significant rise in the ratio of oxycodone mentions to prescriptions written from 1999 through 2001. Although oxycodone prescriptions were written only about a third as often as prescriptions for hydrocodone, emergency room mentions of oxycodone rose to almost the same level as hydrocodone mentions (Zacny et. al. 2003). Although the data reviewed in the report do not distinguish OxyContin from other oxycodone formulations, this trend parallels in time the upsurge of concern regarding OxyContin diversion.

The report reviewed two forms of response that might be brought to bear on the problem. First, drugs can be formulated so as to minimize the likelihood they would be taken for nonmedical effects. Slowing the onset of effects and maintaining steady dose levels both mitigate against the rush of euphoria that opioids can produce. Timed-release formulations provide these features, but the report authors noted that OxyContin's biphasic release method provides a quicker onset of effects than has been typical of gradual-release drug formulations. The other approach is to add an antagonist to the analgesic. The authors admitted the limitations of these narrowly technical recommendations; as they noted, both analgesia and the effects sought by nonmedical users "appear to be mediated through the same neuropharmacological mechanism." Thus, it continues to be the case that the "opioid drugs that are most efficacious in relieving pain also are the opioids with the highest potential for abuse" (Zacny et. al. 2003).

For this reason, the report continued, surveillance, enforcement, education, and prevention remain important. Yet, as the authors noted, a recent program announcement from the National Institute on Drug Abuse seeking proposals to study prevention in this area indicates a lack of consensus on what would be most effective. On the enforcement side, the report noted approvingly the creation of DEA task forces to coordinate with state and local bodies overseeing drug enforcement and medical practice. It emphasized that neither physicians treating pain nor pain patients have played a significant role in opioid diversion.

The task force's report concludes with sweeping calls for more research, including "comprehensive assessment" of nonmedical use. The only policy recommendations call for improved professional education, including rethinking terminology to reduce the tendency to confuse physical dependence (an acceptable side effect for chronic pain patients who need steady, long-term administration of opioid analgesics to control their pain) and addiction (a state with psychological dimensions as well) (Zacny et. al. 2003). These findings and recommendations suggest that, despite decades of research devoted to the search for improved analgesics, little has changed since the

1920s in how the problem is framed. The most significant shift has been to put the needs of pain patients and, by implication, the interests of physicians who treat pain patients at a higher priority level. In calling for "a careful and balanced approach," the task force added to the traditional call for careful controls of drug supplies an appeal not to undertreat pain by denying opioid analgesics to patients who need them.

TREATING PAIN AND TREATING ADDICTION

The treatment of pain as a problem in its own right seemed to some like a retreat to the old-fashioned medicine that focused on alleviating symptoms rather than curing disease. Pain specialists have redefined chronic, intractable pain as a debilitating illness and have developed a range of behavioral, surgical, and pharmacological strategies to help patients cope (Baszanger 1995). These strategies include new regimens and new methods for prescribing opioids, including time-released formulations such as OxyContin. In this context, pain clinics or pain specialists in private practice might well generate seemingly disproportionate numbers of prescriptions for opioids. Unscrupulous physicians could claim to be acting similarly. The increase in prescriptions, as in the past, signaled bad practice to observers and attracted the notice of the DEA, with its standing mission to monitor drug diversion. For pain specialists, news coverage describing their attempts at better pain management as indiscriminate narcotic prescribing seemed a setback.

Analogously, the movement to establish addiction as a treatable disease has meant a struggle to shake the negative image of the addict seeking treatment and to give legitimacy to the new specialty of treating addiction. Physicians seeking to treat opioid addiction outside the highly regulated system of methadone clinics also had to carve out a new professional space in the face of widespread skepticism among their colleagues. They sought to convince the medical profession and society at large that addicts, too, were patients in pain—the psychic pain that drove them to repeated and habit-forming opioid use and the pain of withdrawal that drove them back to the drug. These physicians worked to bring addiction treatment into medical school curricula that had long ignored the problem, founded the American Society of Addiction Medicine, and created the other components of a medical specialty. For them, also, publicity about physicians pandering to deceitful addicts was potentially tarnishing.

At the regulatory level of law, the OxyContin cases created tensions between the Federal Drug Administration (FDA) and the DEA over how deeply implicated the drug itself was in the rising incidence of overdose deaths. The FDA, which had approved OxyContin, had a motive to downplay the responsibility of the manufacturer for misuse and death; its officials argued that in many of the OxyContin cases, the victim had ingested other drugs, like alcohol, that increased the likelihood of death. The DEA, on the other hand, welcomed any evidence that a drug it had classified as dangerous was proving to be so (Meier 2001c, 2002e).

Finally, Purdue and its spokespersons walked a fine line as the company engaged in aggressive damage control. They argued that the company could not have foreseen the problem, based in part on their experience with MS Contin, and at the same time they portrayed drug-seeking addicts as clever criminals who must not be allowed to derail a useful medicine (Udell 2001). Yet this position seems disingenuous. Given the enormous resources that pharmaceutical firms devote to developing and marketing new medications, even a modest investment in anticipating problems might have suggested the likelihood that OxyContin would be misused. The history of the introduction of new psychoactive medications reveals ample precedents. The ease with which the time-release mechanism could be defeated—simply by crushing the pill— should, perhaps, have raised concern. Purdue has embarked on an effort to identify an opioid antagonist that could be added to OxyContin to prevent addicts from experiencing euphoric or withdrawal-relieving effects from the medication; the company estimates that this process will take up to 5 years.

Pharmaceutical research and development has proven particularly adept at producing arrays of drugs with similar, if slightly differing, effects. The ability to patent a new compound, even if it essentially mimics the effects of an already known medication, enables pharmaceutical companies to enter lucrative markets and compete with existing products (Richards n.d.; Peterson 2001). Clearly the challenge of new medications that create new opportunities for street users to obtain illicit drugs will remain with us, and the cat-and-mouse game played by drug users and those who seek to enforce the limits of medically approved use is unlikely to yield a clear victor. However, examining the issue of drug diversion in the United States does provide some basis for understanding how this game has played out.

For example, viewed by seasoned observers of the drug scene, the OxyContin episode is more explicable than media accounts would imply. OxyContin overdoses form part of a larger pattern of opiate overdoses in which heroin and diverted methadone are also implicated (Belluck 2003); in many areas, such as Allegheny County, Pennsylvania, opiate overdose deaths have outnumbered automobile fatalities since about 1999. In research funded by Purdue Pharma, ethnographers analyzed patterns of nonmedical OxyContin use in two Maine cities. They concluded that, far from being an unprecedented and exotic phenomenon, the rash of OxyContin problems was an expectable result of the introduction of a new and powerful opiate into a relatively young and inexperienced population of recreational users (Irwin 2002).

People's ongoing desire to manage their moods, energy levels, and comfort by consuming psychoactive drugs has been increasingly medicalized from the late 19th century to the present. The doctor's office will continue to be a site of negotiation over appropriate means of relieving physical pain and distressing emotional states such as anxiety. Patients' demands are often problematic, as exemplified by requests for antibiotics in cases of viral illness. Their demands are based on expectations promulgated in part by doctors and pharmaceutical manufacturers and in part by a generalized faith in technological progress that characterizes Western culture. America's patchwork of health care coverage and its social service system more generally add to the problem by creating perverse incentives for some patients to seek medications and denying others access to medications they need. Finally, despite scientific medicine's shift to reductionist and somatic therapies and managed care's shortening of the time any patient can spend with a physician, patients still present with "vague complaints" that frequently have a psychological dimension, and they hope their physicians will help them deal with the life issues involved. Physicians too often respond by writing a prescription for an antidepressant or a benzodiazepine.

The regulatory system that categorizes drugs, or contexts of use, as allowable or prohibited is shot through with inconsistencies. Methadone maintenance remains highly regulated in ways that punish and stigmatize patients and limit access to this method of treating opioid addiction; at the same time, nicotine maintenance devices for would-be ex-smokers, which operate on the same principle of maintaining the addiction at a stable dose level, are widely and legally hawked. Some drugs remain locked on the wrong side of the divide, although the evidence of their uselessness as medications is not clear. State-level initiatives to approve marijuana for medical use, and attempts to study marijuana as medicine, have alarmed the federal drug policy establishment; the DEA has threatened to prosecute any physician prescribing marijuana under such state authorization and recently arrested two people in California for growing marijuana intended for medical use. As Lasagna (1965) has written, the banning of heroin in the United States is not a serious loss, given its similarity of effects to morphine, but:

> [If] it *were* a serious loss, it would be almost impossible ... to reintroduce the drug into medical usage because of the real or imagined conflict of such usage with the goals of law enforcement officers whose eyes are focused on the eradication of the illegal use of heroin by addicts, and because of the horrible but ill-deserved reputation the drug has acquired over the years.

Media treatment of these issues, like its coverage of illicit drug use more generally, remains unguided by historical memory and unchastened by criticism. Every drug "epidemic" hits the headlines as if it were a new and unique threat. The polity is left without effective information or guidance about how to assess problems arising from psychoactive drug use. To quote Lasagna (1965): "The likelihood of coming up with ... solutions [to the problem of drug diversion] will probably be inversely proportional to the distortions and lack of perspective in the picture we draw of the addict and of the addiction problem." I would add that we must also better understand what kinds of relief patients seek when they consult physicians and what people of all kinds expect when they take psychoactive drugs.

REFERENCES

Acker CJ. Addiction and the laboratory: the work of the National Research Council's Committee on Drug Addiction, 1928–1939. *Isis* 1995a; 86:167–193.

Acker CJ. From all purpose anodyne to marker of deviance: physicians' attitudes toward opiates in the U.S., 1890–1940. In: Porter R, Teich M (Eds). *Drugs and Narcotics in History*. Cambridge: Cambridge University Press, 1995b, pp 114–132.

Acker CJ. Planning and serendipity in the search for a nonaddicting opiate analgesic. In: Higby GJ, Stroud EC (Eds). *The Inside Story of Medicines: A Symposium*. Madison: American Institute for the History of Pharmacy, 1997, pp 139–157.

Acker CJ. *Creating the American Junkie: Addiction Research in the Classic Era of Narcotic Control*. Baltimore: Johns Hopkins University Press, 2001.

Acker CJ. Portrait of an addicted family: dynamics of opiate addiction in the early twentieth century. In: Tracy SW, Acker CJ, (Eds). *Altering American Consciousness: Essays on the History of Alcohol and Drug Use in the United States, 1800–2000*. Amherst: University of Massachusetts Press, in press.

American Medical Association. *Nostrums and Quackery and Pseudo-Medicine*, Vol. 1. Chicago: Press of the American Medical Association, 1911.

American Medical Association. *Nostrums and Quackery and Pseudo-Medicine*, Vol. 2. Chicago: Press of the American Medical Association, 1921.

American Medical Association. *Nostrums and Quackery and Pseudo-Medicine*, Vol. 3. Chicago: Press of the American Medical Association, 1936.

Anthony JC. The regulation of dangerous psychoactive drugs. In: Morgan JP, Kagan DV (Eds). *Society and Medication: Conflicting Signals for Prescribers and Patients*. Lexington, MA: Lexington Books, 1983, 163–180.

Baszanger I. *Inventing Pain Medicine: From the Laboratory to the Clinic*. New Brunswick: Rutgers University Press, 1995.

Belluck P. Methadone, once the way out, suddenly grows as a killer drug. *New York Times*, national ed. 2003; February 9:A1, A20.

Courtwright DT. *Dark Paradise: Opiate Addiction in America before 1940*. Cambridge: Harvard University Press, 1982.

Courtwright DT. *Forces of Habit: Drugs and the Making of the Modern World*. Cambridge: Harvard University Press, 2001.

Eddy NB. *The National Research Council Involvement in the Opiate Problem, 1928–1971*. Washington, DC: National Academy of Sciences, 1973.

Gellman M, Ciancutti CJ. Toxic levels of diazepam explain mysterious boot Lude overdoses. *Street Pharmacologist* 1980; 3:8–9.

Howard-Jones N. A critical study of the origins and early development of hypodermic medication. *J Hist Med Allied Sci* 1947; 2:201–245.

Irwin K. Placing OxyContin use in context: report from Maine. *Taking Drug Users Seriously: Fourth National Harm Reduction Conference.* Seattle, 2002.

Kleinman A. *The Illness Narratives: Suffering, Healing and the Human Condition.* New York: Basic Books, 1988.

Lasagna L. Addicting drugs and medical practice: toward the elaboration of realistic goals and the eradication of myths, mirages, and half-truths. In: Wilner DM, Kassebaum GG (Eds). *Narcotics.* New York: McGraw-Hill, 1965, pp 53–66.

McAllister WB. *Drug Diplomacy in the Twentieth Century: An International History.* New York: Routledge, 2000.

Meier B. Maker chose not to use a drug abuse safeguard. *New York Times,* national ed. 2001a; August 13:A11.

Meier B. At painkiller trouble spot, signs seen as alarming didn't alarm drug's maker. *New York Times,* national ed. 2001b; December 10:A16.

Meier B. Official faults drug company for marketing of its painkiller. *New York Times,* national ed. 2001c; December 12:A16.

Meier B. OxyContin prescribers face charges in fatal overdoses. *New York Times,* national ed. 2002a; January 19:A12.

Meier B. A small-town clinic looms large as a top source of disputed painkillers. *New York Times,* national ed. 2002b; February 10:18.

Meier B. Closing arguments made in trial of doctor in OxyContin deaths. *New York Times,* national ed. 2002c; February 19:A16.

Meier B. Doctor is sentenced for OxyContin deaths. *New York Times,* national ed. 2002d; March 23:A11.

Meier B. OxyContin deaths said to be up sharply. *New York Times,* national ed. 2002e; April 15:A14.

Morgan JP. Preface and acknowledgments. In: Morgan JP, Kagan DV (Eds). *Society and Medication: Conflicting Signals for Prescribers and Patients.* Lexington, MA: Lexington Books, 1983.

Morgan JP, Kagan DV. The dusting of America: the image of phencyclidine (PCP) in the popular media. In: Smith DE, Wesson D, Buxton M, et al. (Eds). *PCP: Problems and Prevention.* San Francisco: Haight Ashbury, 1982, pp 11–20.

Musto DF. *The American Disease: Origins of Narcotic Control.* New Haven: Yale University Press, 1973.

Passe L. Street talk: pill pourri. *Street Pharmacologist* 1981; 4:6.

Pawlak V. Street talk. *Street Pharmacologist* 1980; 3:11.

Peterson M. New medicines seldom contain anything new, study finds. *New York Times,* national ed. 2001; May 29:C1, 8.

Richards AN. *Alfred Newton Richards Papers,* Archives of the University of Pennsylvania, Philadelphia, Box 11, Folder 41, n.d. (ca. 1930).

Rosenberg CE. The therapeutic revolution: medicine, meaning, and social change in nineteenth-century America. In: Rosenberg CE, Vogel MJ (Eds). *The Therapeutic Revolution: Essays in the Social History of American Medicine.* Philadelphia: University of Pennsylvania Press, 1979.

Tomes N. *The Gospel of Germs: Men, Women, and the Microbe in American Life.* Cambridge: Harvard University Press, 1998.

Tough P. The OxyContin underground. *New York Times Magazine* 2001; July 29:32.

Udell HR. Letter to editor. *New York Times Magazine* 2001; August 5:8.

Zacny J, Bigelow G, Compton P, et al. College on Problems of Drug Dependence taskforce on prescription opioid non-medical use and abuse: position statement. *Drug Alcohol Depend* 2003; 69:215–232.

Zinberg NE. *Drug, Set, and Setting: The Basis for Controlled Intoxicant Use.* New Haven: Yale University Press, 1984.

Correspondence to: Caroline Jean Acker, PhD, Department of History, Baker Hall 240, Carnegie Mellon University, Pittsburgh, PA 15213–3890, USA. Email: acker@andrew.cmu.edu.

Opioids and Pain Relief: A Historical Perspective,
Progress in Pain Research and Management, Vol.
25, edited by Marcia L. Meldrum, IASP Press,
Seattle, © 2003.

5

Analgesic Research at the National Institutes of Health: State of the Art 1930s to the Present

Kenner C. Rice

*Laboratory of Medicinal Chemistry, National Institute of Diabetes
and Digestive and Kidney Diseases, National Institutes of Health,
Department of Health and Human Services, Bethesda, Maryland, USA*

This chapter presents an overview, from a medicinal chemistry perspective, of the development of the analgesic program at the U.S. National Institutes of Health (NIH) from its predecessor begun under the auspices of the National Academy of Sciences in 1929, and reviews highlights of some of the important discoveries during this period. The following overlapping research themes are discussed: the search for a nonaddicting analgesic, the development of a practical chemical synthesis of morphine and related drugs independent of the opium poppy, and the production of novel drugs, both as clinically useful medications and as research tools for neuroscience and addiction research. The work of the analgesic program has resulted in the development of a broad array of drugs, with vastly different pharmacological profiles that are useful in diverse areas, which range from animal studies to identify drug recognition sites (receptors) to measurement of drug receptors in conscious humans and to the clinical treatment of pain and narcotic addiction. These novel drugs include opioid agonists (which produce morphine-like actions), antagonists (antidotes that reverse or prevent the actions of agonists), and agonist-antagonists (which combine these two kinds of actions in the same drug). The ramifications of these discoveries in the broader context of our developing understanding of opioid abuse and treatment and the opioid receptor-endorphin system are discussed. Some of the principal investigators involved in the NIH analgesic program are shown in Figs. 1–7.

THE BEGINNING

The NIH analgesic program evolved from the activities of the New York City Bureau of Social Hygiene, originated in 1913 by John D. Rockefeller, Jr. The bureau created the Committee on Drug Addiction in 1921 to deal with drug abuse problems. The bureau initiated discussion with the National Research Council (NRC), part of the National Academy of Sciences (NAS), which in 1928 resulted in the establishment of the Temporary Advisory Committee on Drug Addiction of the NRC Division of Medical Sciences (DMS). William C. White, then chair of the DMS, became chair of the advisory committee, which had 10 members in addition to White, including the eminent pharmacologist Reid Hunt of Harvard Medical School (Eddy 1973; May and Jacobson 1989; Acker 2001). During planning of the program on opiate analgesics on January 12, 1929, Hunt articulated a guiding premise for the program: "A thorough study of the morphine molecule might show a possibility of separating the analgesic form from the habit forming property ... work along these lines would involve cooperation between the highest type of organic chemists and pharmacologists" (White 1941; Eddy 1973). Hunt further pointed out that the need for cocaine had declined after the discovery of procaine (Novocain) and that a similar reduction in medical requirements for morphine might be achieved with the introduction of synthetic analgesics.

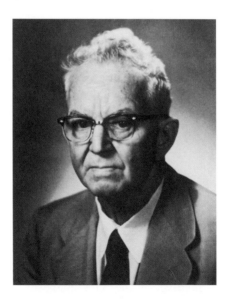

Fig. 1, Dr, Lyndon F. Small.

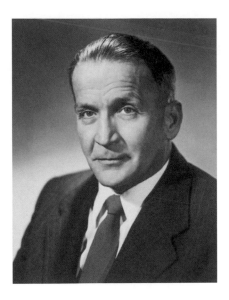

Fig. 2. Dr. Erich Mosettig.

MORPHINE AND PHENANTHRENE DERIVATIVES AT THE UNIVERSITY OF VIRGINIA

The committee recognized that basic research was essential to accomplishing the goal of developing improved analgesics and established three collaborating programs in organic chemistry, pharmacology, and clinical testing. Lyndon F. Small (Fig. 1) began the chemistry program at the University of Virginia in Charlottesville in 1929 and recruited Erich Mosettig (Fig. 2) from the laboratory of the eminent Austrian chemist Ernest Späth as his assistant (Eddy 1973). The pharmacology program began under Nathan B. Eddy (Fig. 3) at the University of Michigan in Ann Arbor in 1930. Clifton K. Himmelsbach (Fig. 4) began the clinical program in temporary quarters at the Federal Penitentiary at Fort Leavenworth, Kansas, and soon transferred to the Addiction Research Center of the U.S. Public Health Service in Lexington, Kentucky, after its opening in May 1935. The University of Virginia provided laboratory space for Small and Mosettig, who together with their students and Mrs. Small as secretary formed the Drug Addiction Laboratory (Mosettig 1959; Eddy 1973).

The committee decided that one of its initial steps should be a complete survey of the chemistry and pharmacology of the opium alkaloids and derivatives. Small, assisted by Robert Lutz of the University of Virginia, published the first complete review of the chemistry of the opium alkaloids, containing approximately 2,100 references (Small 1932). The existing

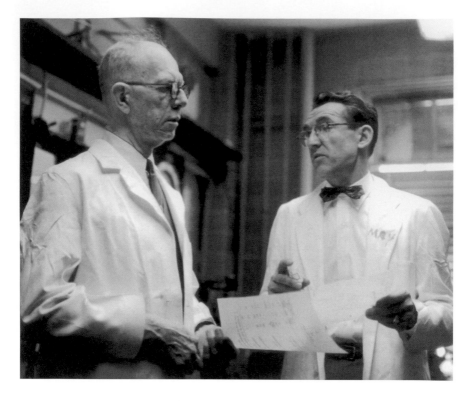

Fig. 3. Dr. Nathan B. Eddy and Dr. Everette L. May.

pharmacological work on the opium alkaloids consisted of more than 9,100 references and was reviewed in two parts, published in the early 1940s: (1) the pharmacology of morphine (Krueger et al. 1941), and (2) that of other alkaloids and derivatives (Krueger et al. 1943). Small organized the chemical program into two arms. In the first set of studies, he concentrated on the chemistry of the morphine alkaloids and the modification of functional groups present in these molecules. Mosettig meanwhile pursued the second approach of total synthesis of improved analgesics from simple, inactive ring systems by addition of some of the functional groups present in the morphine molecule. One of the templates selected for these studies was phenanthrene, because morphine was (correctly) thought to contain a hydrophenanthrene skeleton. Evidence for this structural feature partly resulted from the phenanthrene derivatives that had appeared in the degradative studies during the structural elucidation of the morphine alkaloids. These and other studies (Small 1932; Holmes 1952) led to Gulland and Robinson's formulation of the structure of morphine and thebaine in 1925. Although these structures were not universally accepted as correct at the time, Small elected to base his studies on them when he began his work in the Drug Addiction Laboratory only 4 years later. This decision placed Small in an advantageous position because Gulland and Robinson's formulations were finally proven correct in 1952 by the first unequivocal total synthesis of morphine and codeine (Gates and Tschudi 1952, 1956).

The compounds synthesized by Small and Mosettig's groups were initially studied in animal assays by Eddy and his associates at Michigan. They employed seven quantitative pharmacological assays to measure the major effects of morphine recognized at the time and classified the results for each compound according to six chemical changes in the morphine molecule (Small et al. 1938). Himmelsbach and his associates then evaluated selected drugs for their ability to substitute for morphine in dependent human subjects and for their ability to maintain dependence in these subjects after morphine was discontinued. An interim report (Small et al. 1938) provided numerous animal data and results on 16 compounds studied in humans.

By the end of the first 10 years of the program, Small and his team had designed and synthesized nearly 500 compounds for pharmacological study (White 1941; May and Jacobson 1989). They used a systematic medicinal chemical approach, relating molecular structure to pharmacological activity at each step. First, they prepared pure samples of morphine, codeine, and other known compounds as pharmacological standards. The relationship of each of the functional groups in the morphine molecule to activity was then

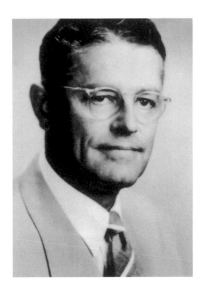

Fig. 4. Dr. Clifton K. Himmelsbach.

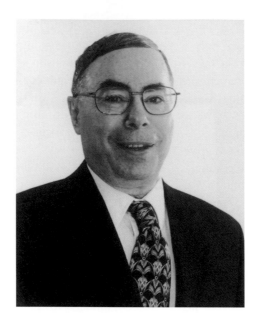

Fig. 5. Dr. Arthur E. Jacobson.

assessed by synthesis and pharmacological study of the appropriate compounds. Small and his associates clearly recognized that alterations in chemical structure could result in often predictable changes in pharmacological
profile. He and his group also found that appropriate structural changes
either increased or decreased desirable pharmacological properties of novel
compounds relative to standard drugs. These studies provided the foundation of modern structure-activity relationships in the opiate series. This program was truly state of the art in all respects, and was, in my opinion, well
ahead of its time.

Small's systematic chemical investigations resulted in many publications on the fundamental chemistry of the morphine alkaloids and the identification of several important new compounds (Small et al. 1938; White
1941; Mosettig 1959; Newman et al. 1992). He synthesized C-ring isomers
of codeine and morphine, their dihydro derivatives, and halogenomorphides
and codides. Small prepared 4-hydroxy derivatives in which the oxide bridge
in the morphine alkaloids was opened. He studied the complex reduction of
thebaine and prepared desoxycodeine and morphine derivatives. He also
isolated crystalline neopine methyl ether among the products from catalytic
reduction of thebaine.

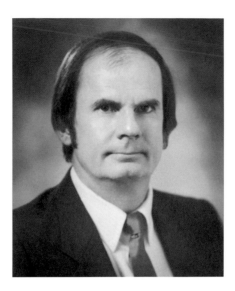

Fig. 6. Dr. Kenner C. Rice.

Small investigated the chemistry of 14-hydroxycodeinone and its derivatives; these include the clinically valuable 14-hydroxydihydrocodeinone (oxycodone), which was the second most widely used opioid analgesic in U.S. medicine in 2002. His work on the separation and characterization of the phenyldihydrothebaines and their transformation products would ultimately lead to the elucidation of their structure after more than 40 years of study.

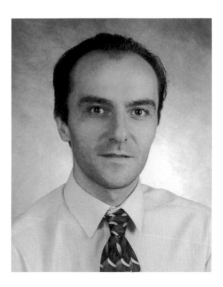

Fig. 7. Dr. Andrew Coop.

Small also studied the action of organometallic reagents on a number of opium derivatives; this work led him to the synthesis of metopon. In his pivotal 1936 paper, he showed that 8,14-dihydrothebaine reacts with methylmagnesium iodide to give principally 5-methyldihydrothebainone; upon further transformation, this material provided 5-methyldihydromorphinone, also known as metopon (Small et al. 1936). Extensive study of metopon (Fig. 8) in animals and later in humans showed that the compound retained strong morphine-like analgesia but caused fewer undesirable side effects than morphine. These observations validated Hunt's basic premise that specific chemical modification of the morphine molecule might separate the beneficial and detrimental effects of morphine; the results with metopon were the long-sought "proof of principle" that still permeates contemporary opioid research. Other compounds with differential properties such as desomorphine (Fig. 8) also emerged from Small's program. Desomorphine was ultimately characterized as a potent, rapid, and short-acting analgesic, but it offered no advantages over morphine.

Small received numerous scientific honors during his career. He (jointly with Eddy) was the first recipient of the American Pharmaceutical Association Scientific Award presented on June 27, 1939 by Harry Anslinger, Commissioner of the Bureau of Narcotics of the U.S. Treasury Department (Eddy 1973). On the basis of his work in opiate chemistry, Small was elected to the National Academy of Sciences in 1941 and received the Hillebrand Prize of the Washington Section of the American Chemical Society in 1949 (Mosettig 1959). His program greatly expanded alkaloid research in the United States and stimulated structure-activity studies. He trained many postdoctoral fellows, among these the late Henry Rapoport, one of the greatest organic chemists of our time. Small was the editor-in-chief of the *Journal of Organic Chemistry* from 1938 to 1951. He served in many other prestigious elected and appointed posts during his career including Chief of the Laboratory of Chemistry, National Institute of Arthritis and Metabolic Diseases (1951–1957), succeeding Claude S. Hudson. Small was a superb microanalyst and brilliant experimentalist (Mosettig 1959).

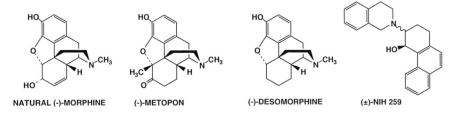

Fig. 8. Structures of natural (−)-morphine, (−)-metopon, (−)-desomorphine, and (±)-NIH 259.

Mosettig and his associates systematically developed many new compounds and published numerous papers on their synthetic derivatives based on the phenanthrene, benzofuran, and carbazole ring systems (White 1941). They explored and expanded the chemistry of these ring systems, producing numerous derivatives for Eddy to evaluate. Morphine was considered to be both an isoquinoline and a phenanthrene derivative containing a secondary alcohol, a tertiary amine, and a phenolic hydroxyl function. These functional groups, alone or in combination, were appended to the basic ring systems, with amino-containing side chains being frequently incorporated in the target compounds. One of the most notable compounds developed by Mosettig and his group was 3-[2-(1,2,3,4-tetrahydroisoquinolinolyl)]-4-hydroxy-1,2,3,4-tetrahydrophenanthrene (NIH 259, Fig. 8). In assays, this derivative showed analgesic activity approaching that of codeine and did not support morphine addiction in dependent human subjects (Small 1937). Studies with this compound ended after an unexplained toxic reaction was observed (Eddy 1973).

The final report of the Committee on Drug Addiction, published by White under the auspices of the NRC in 1941, contained reprints of 153 chemical, pharmacological, and clinical papers published during 1930–1941. Results during this period were summarized by Eddy, Mosettig, and Small as follows:

> The systematic scientific program has resulted in the accumulation of much affirmative data on two major problems: First, the quantitative dissociation of the complex morphine effect on the living organism by chemical modification of the morphine molecule; and second, the development of compounds with definite analgesic action by suitable chemical additions to simple nuclei. (White 1941)

In 1938, Small, Mosettig, and Eddy accepted invitations to move their programs to the National Institute of Health (then a single institute) under government sponsorship, and in 1939, the researchers arrived at the NIH facility at 25th and E Streets in Washington, DC. When Building 4 opened on the main NIH campus in Bethesda, Maryland, Small, Mosettig, and their associates moved there to their permanent quarters in May, 1941 (Eddy 1973). Eddy began his work in Building 2 in Bethesda and later joined Small and Mosettig.

During World War II, an Advisory Committee on Drug Addiction appointed by Lewis H. Weed, chair of the DMS, served to provide advice on matters pertaining to opiate drugs. In 1947, Weed established the larger Committee on Drug Addiction and Narcotics (CDAN) to serve this function. CDAN became the Committee on Problems of Drug Dependence (CPDD) in 1967 (Eddy 1973). In 1976, the CPDD became an independent entity.

Reorganized into a membership group in 1991, the committee was renamed the College on Problems of Drug Dependence. An excellent review of the history of the CPDD (May and Jacobson 1989) serves to summarize and update the earlier account describing events from 1929 to 1971 (Eddy 1973). Arthur E. Jacobson (Fig. 5) and I (Fig. 6) reviewed the evolution of the NIH analgesic program to the contemporary Laboratory of Medicinal Chemistry as part of the National Institute of Diabetes and Digestive and Kidney Diseases (NIDDK) and its relationship with the CPDD on the 50th anniversary of its beginning in Bethesda (Jacobson and Rice 1992).

NIH RESEARCH ON BENZOMORPHANS, PHENYLMORPHANS, METHADONE DERIVATIVES, AND CANNABINOIDS

Everette L. May, a young scientist from the University of Virginia, joined Small's group in Bethesda on December 1, 1941. May (Fig. 3) had received his Ph.D. at the University of Virginia in 1939 working under Mosettig on the analgesic program (May 1939). With the coming of World War II, the major emphasis in the laboratory shifted to antimalarial research because of anticipated quinine shortages. One compound from this program, 3-bromo-N,N-diheptylaminomethyl-phenanthrene-10-methanol, emerged as a life-saving drug during the Vietnam War for treatment of malaria infections resistant to standard therapy (May 1992).

The end of the war saw a renewed focus on the analgesic program. At NIH, Small continued his investigations of the morphine alkaloids while May and Mosettig began their studies on methadone, isomethadone, 3-hydroxy-N-methylmorphinan, and other derivatives that had been developed in Germany and Switzerland during the war. They synthesized and pharmacologically evaluated all the possible methadols and isomethadols and their O-acetyl derivatives (May 1992). During this work, May synthesized LAAM (levo-α-acetylmethadol), an orally active, longer acting, and more potent drug than methadone that is now used in maintenance therapy of recovering heroin addicts.

In the mid 1950s, May made additional major discoveries when he synthesized the 6,7-benzomorphans as a potential novel class of analgesics and then developed the 5-phenylmorphans. He hypothesized that molecules smaller and chemically simpler than morphine might have more favorable properties as long as they retained the N-methyl and the quaternary carbon atom believed at the time to be essential for strong analgesic activity, and tested his idea by dissecting the morphine molecule (as shown in Fig. 9) into these two new types of compounds (May 1992). May and his associates at NIH developed the structure-activity relationships in the benzomorphan series extensively (May and Eddy 1969); these studies were extended in numerous laboratories worldwide (Palmer and Strauss 1977).

This small-molecule work provided many valuable research tools for elucidation of the opioid receptor–endorphin system. Among these are SKF 10,047, an opioid antagonist; cyclazocine, an agonist-antagonist; and bremazocine, an agonist; as well as the better-known drugs phenazocine and pentazocine. Phenazocine (Prinadol, Narphen, NIH 7519), originated by May and associates, was formerly prescribed in the United States and Europe as a potent analgesic. Pentazocine (Talwin), a benzomorphan agonist-antagonist with less dependence liability (Schedule 4) than morphine, was developed by Sterling-Winthrop. The first agonist-antagonist marketed as an analgesic and the vanguard of this class of drugs for the treatment of pain, pentazocine is still prescribed in the United States and other countries for moderate pain. Structures of some of these compounds are shown in Fig. 10.

The introduction of the benzomorphans as analgesics by May, followed by a landmark paper (Archer et al. 1964) on the effect of the *N*-substituent in the benzomorphan series, as well as the development of pentazocine greatly advanced and stimulated research on the agonist-antagonist approach to the development of pain medications. These events influenced the introduction of nalbuphine, butorphanol, and buprenorphine as clinically useful analgesics. Buprenorphine has recently received approval from the U.S. Food and Drug Administration for treatment of heroin dependence.

After Eddy's retirement in 1960, May replaced him as section chief and changed the name of the Analgesics Section to the Section on Medicinal Chemistry. Eddy continued in his role as pharmacologist and as biological

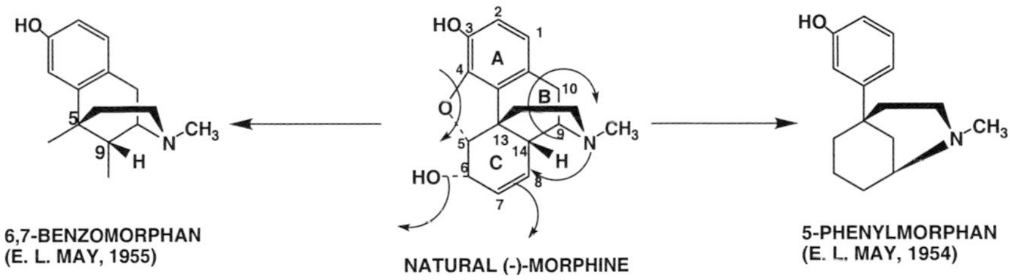

6,7-BENZOMORPHAN
(E. L. MAY, 1955)

NATURAL (-)-MORPHINE

5-PHENYLMORPHAN
(E. L. MAY, 1954)

Fig. 9. May's conceptualization of the 6,7-benzomorphans and the 5-phenylmorphans. The 6,7-benzomorphans are derived from morphine by removal of the oxide bridge and carbon atoms 6 and 7 to open the C ring and provide the C-5 and C-9 methyl groups in the benzomorphan structure. The 5-phenylmorphans are derived from morphine by removal of the oxide bridge and the C-6 hydroxyl group, reduction of the 7,8-double bond, removal of carbon atoms 9 and 10, and relocation of the nitrogen atom to the C-8 position of morphine.

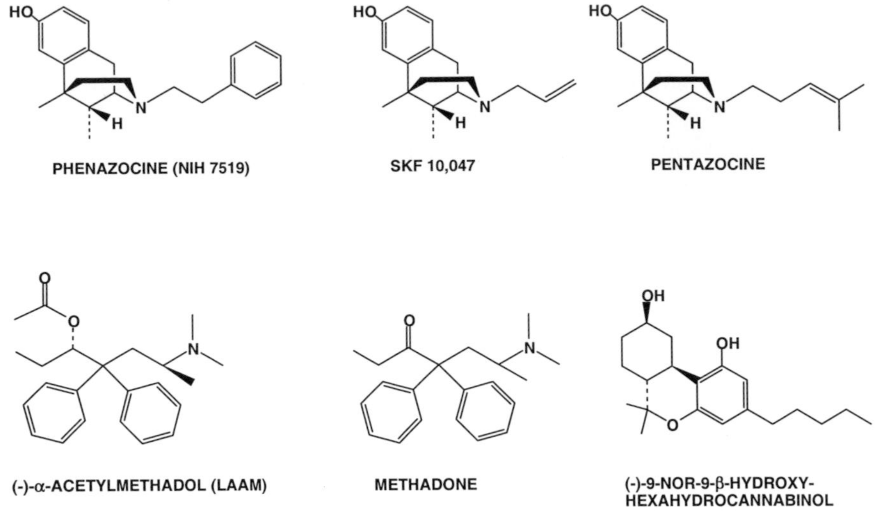

PHENAZOCINE (NIH 7519)   SKF 10,047   PENTAZOCINE

(-)-α-ACETYLMETHADOL (LAAM)   METHADONE   (-)-9-NOR-9-β-HYDROXY-
                                                       HEXAHYDROCANNABINOL

Fig. 10. Structures of phenazocine, SKF 10,047, pentazocine, levo-α-acetylmethadol (LAAM), methadone, and (–)-9-nor-9β-hydroxyhexahydrocannabinol.

coordinator of the CPDD until 1967, when May assumed the biological coordinator duties.

In the early 1970s, May and Raymond Wilson (a postdoctoral fellow from the University of Kansas) began a program on the cannabinoids that led to the discovery of the cannabinoid receptors. Their critical finding was that (–)-9-nor-9β-hydroxyhexahydrocannabinol (Fig. 10) demonstrated morphine-like analgesic potency in animal tests while the racemic α and β compounds showed strong cannabinoid properties (Wilson and May 1976). Subsequent studies with the (–)-9β compound established that this compound did not act via the opioid receptors (Johnson and Milne 1981). Based on this critical differentiation of the 9β compound from the opioids, M.R. Johnson initiated a comprehensive synthetic program on cannabinoids at Pfizer. This work provided the compounds that made it possible for A.C. Howlett, Johnson, and their associates to publish the biochemical identification of the cannabinoid receptor (Devane et al. 1988).

Definitive autoradiographic studies, conducted by Miles Herkenham in collaboration with Johnson, Brian de Costa, then a postdoctoral fellow in my research group, and myself, used the Pfizer drug [³H]CP55,940 to reveal the anatomical distribution of the brain cannabinoid receptor in several species, including humans. The anatomical findings explained the almost complete lack of acute cannabinoid toxicity (Herkenham et al. 1990). These autoradiographic studies were also central to Lisa Matsuda's identification of the newly cloned cannabinoid receptor at NIH (Matsuda et al. 1990). These advances continue to have highly significant ramifications in the study of the central nervous system (CNS), in research on drug abuse and addiction, and in contemporary medicinal chemistry, and can be traced to the original work of May and Wilson.

Like Small, May has received many forms of professional recognition during his long and still active career at the Virginia Commonwealth University/Medical College of Virginia (VCU/MCV) in Richmond. These include the 1968 Hillebrand Award (jointly with Eddy) of the Washington Chemical Society, the 1976 American Pharmaceutical Association Research Achievement Award in Medicinal and Pharmaceutical Chemistry, the 1979 American Chemical Society E.E. Smissman Award in Medicinal Chemistry (May 1980), the 1981 Nathan B. Eddy Award of the Committee on Problems of Drug Dependence (May 1982), and the 1992 American Chemical Society Alfred Burger Award in Medicinal Chemistry (May 1992). He was appointed to honorary membership in the Japanese Pharmaceutical Society in 1992, an honor conferred upon few individuals outside Japan.

UNNATURAL OPIATES AND THE NIH
OPIATE TOTAL SYNTHESIS

It was my good fortune to join May's group (the Section on Medicinal Chemistry, NIDDK) on June 26, 1974, and play a part in this program as one of his last postdoctoral fellows at NIH. Many studies were in progress during this exciting period to further characterize the newly discovered opioid receptor (then singular). Since then, diverse lines of investigation have provided much insight into the opioid receptor-endorphin system. Three types of opioid receptor (μ, δ, and κ) have been identified and cloned, and numerous peptides (endorphins) that function as endogenous ligands for the receptors have been identified and characterized (Akil, this volume). This system plays a central role in modulating normal mammalian function and behavior and mediates the effects of opioid drugs and their antagonists. Morphine, the prototypic opioid agonist, acts principally through the μ-opioid receptor. Dysfunction of the opioid receptor system has been linked to a number of central and peripheral disorders. The μ, δ, and κ receptors exhibit high-affinity binding for many drugs in the low nanomolar range and are localized in discrete brain regions in order to serve specific functions. The receptors recognize mirror image forms (enantiomers) of drugs differently; these drugs thus exhibit enantioselectivity in binding and in vivo effects.

    One of my first projects in May's group was the chemical synthesis of
viable quantities of unnatural (+)-enantiomers (mirror image forms) of natural codeine and morphine. Mario Aceto at VCU/MCV had suggested the
synthesis of these compounds for pharmacological evaluation during his
discussions with Louis Harris (then chair of the MCV pharmacology department) and May. At that time, no suitable methodology existed for the practical total synthesis of the required amounts of these unnatural mirror-image
variants. Goto and Yamamoto had earlier described a semisynthetic, low-
yielding route to these compounds from the alkaloid (–)-sinomenine (May
1992). Through the generosity of Mikio Takeda of Tanabe Laboratories in
Japan, May procured 50 g of (–)-sinomenine as starting material, and work on
the synthesis project began on March 2, 1976 (Fig. 11). Ikuo Iijima, a visiting
scientist from Tanabe and a superb organic chemist and experimentalist,
extensively modified and improved the original route to these targets and
synthesized the (+)-enantiomers of natural (–)-morphine and (–)-codeine
(Iijima et al. 1977).

    Later, Iijima also synthesized about 1 g of (+)-naloxone (Iijima et al.
1978), the previously unknown enantiomer of the clinically used opioid
antagonist (Narcan, Figs. 11 and 12). We showed that these (+)-enantiomers
had 1,000- to 10,000-fold less activity than their naturally derived counter-
parts (Jacquet et al. 1977). These unnatural enantiomers and some of their
chemical intermediates such as (+)-oxymorphone have proved (Rice 1985a)

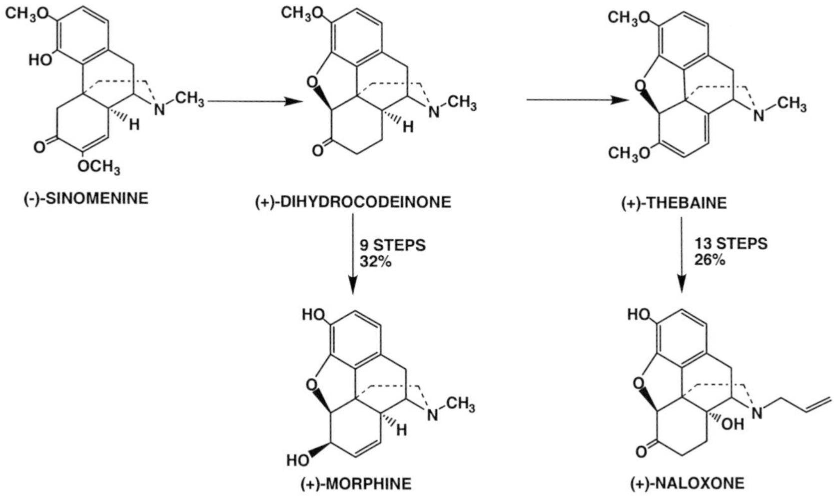

Fig. 11. Chemical synthesis of unnatural (+)-morphine and (+)-naloxone from
(–)-sinomenine.

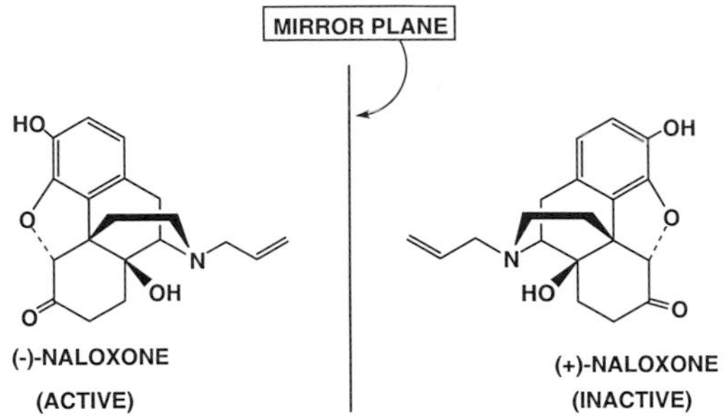

Fig. 12. (–)-Naloxone (Narcan) and the inactive (+)-enantiomer.

to be valuable research tools for the detection and characterization of opioid receptor-mediated effects.

During the 1970s, our group and a number of others internationally initiated projects to develop a practical total synthesis of opium alkaloids. Chief among the factors motivating our work at NIH were a worldwide opium shortage in 1973–1975 (Schwartz 1980), the unavailability of sinomenine as starting material, and the research requirements for larger quantities of (+)-naloxone and new compounds in the unnatural opiate series.

Upon May's retirement from NIH in February 1977, Arnold Brossi became chief of the Section on Medicinal Chemistry with the permanent senior staff consisting of Arthur E. Jacobson and myself. Jacobson succeeded May as biological coordinator of the Drug Testing Program of the CPDD. In 1987, Jacobson and I joined the Laboratory of Neuroscience (headed by Phil Skolnick), and I was named chief of the Section on Drug Design and Synthesis. Subsequently, I became chief of the contemporary Laboratory of Medicinal Chemistry, which was established in 1989.

The section began its work on the total synthesis of morphine alkaloids in the late 1970s. The first approach attempted at NIH was a biomimetic route involving the oxidation of reticuline derivatives to morphinan precursors of the natural alkaloids. We developed an excellent route to the enantiomers of norreticuline, reticuline (Rice and Brossi 1980), pavine, and isopavine derivatives (Rice et al. 1980) utilizing unprotected phenolic intermediates. However, we were unable to identify a practical method by which to convert norreticuline or its derivatives to morphine alkaloids. In other analgesic work during this period, Brossi and associates synthesized numerous ketomorphinans and summarized their findings (Schmidhammer et al. 1983).

Soon afterward, I initiated a conceptually different approach to the practical total synthesis of the morphine alkaloids, which proved quite successful (Rice 1980, 1983, 1985a). This route utilized unprotected phenolic intermediates and used a modified Grewe cyclization to form the morphine carbon-nitrogen skeleton, and also employed novel oxide bridge closure in the *N*-nor series. The critical cyclization was initially successful on January 22, 1979, and I first published the new synthetic method, now known as the NIH opiate total synthesis (Fig. 13), in 1980 (Rice 1980). Later I extended and refined the method to give either the natural or unnatural opiate enantiomers (Rice 1983, 1985a,b, 1986). We have repeated the synthesis many times in the laboratory, using commercially available starting materials to prepare more than 100 g of chiral, correctly oxygenated morphinan intermediates in each batch.

We later increased the versatility of the NIH opiate total synthesis route by adapting this process to the *N*-nor series (Rice and Newman 1997), which allowed us to make a highly efficient sequential conversion of

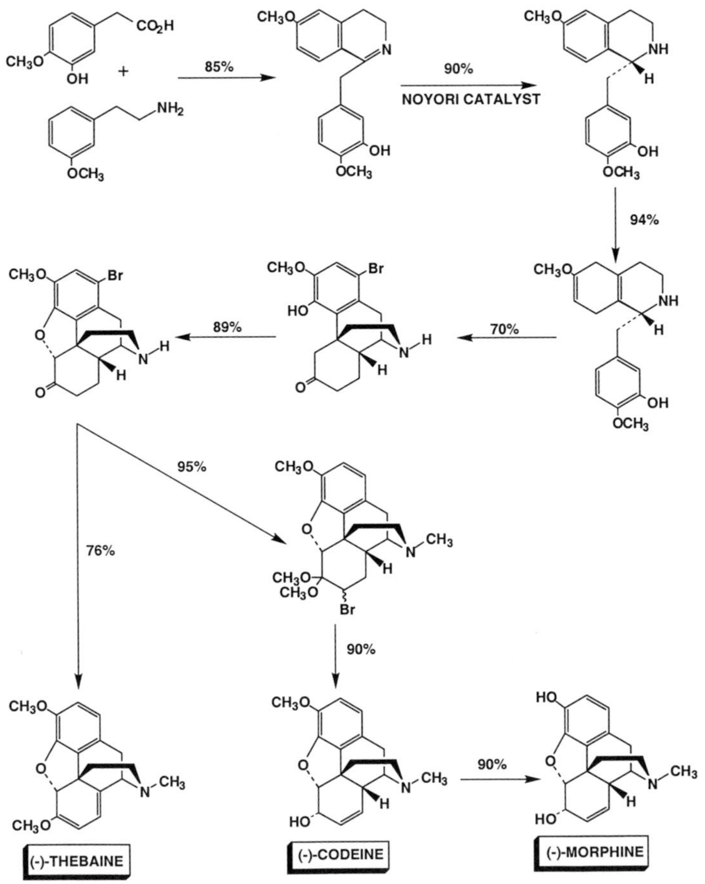

Fig. 13. The NIH opiate total synthesis showing the isolated intermediates.

1-bromonordihydrothebainone to nordihydrocodeinone, northebaine, noroxy-codone, and noroxymorphone and to simplify substantially the total synthesis of the thebaine-based drugs. Because the pharmacological profile of drugs in the opiate series is largely determined by the nitrogen substituent, this methodology expanded the number and diversity of synthetic products. We were able to employ various N-nor intermediates as starting material for many drugs, including the medically important N-methyl derivatives. The overall chemical yield of codeine, morphine, and thebaine from commercially available materials is 32–37%, with only 5–7 isolated (filtered and washed) intermediates.

The route has been utilized to prepare numerous unnatural opium derivatives and is presently under development as a manufacturing process for the total synthesis of opium-derived medical narcotics and their antagonists. The NIH opiate total synthesis constitutes the only practical methodology available for this purpose. This method offers unlimited production of all opium-derived narcotic agonists and antagonists independent of foreign sources of opium, renders the unnatural isomers of the same compounds equally available as drugs and research tools, and offers the prospect of eradicating opium poppy cultivation and thus, eventually, illicit heroin production (Rice 2002).

HIGHLY SELECTIVE OPIOID RECEPTOR AFFINITY LABELS, PURIFICATION OF THE DELTA OPIOID RECEPTOR, AND DELTA RECEPTOR AGONISTS

Concurrently with the work on the opiate total synthesis, we began a program to develop affinity labels as research tools for the opioid receptor subtypes. We introduced the isothiocyanate function to develop highly selective affinity ligands (Fig. 14) to label the μ-, δ-, and κ-opioid receptors (Rice et al. 1983; de Costa et al. 1989). These affinity ligands proved to be valuable research tools for further elucidation of the receptor structure and function. In one example, we designed and synthesized (+)-cis-superfit based on the ultra-potent (+)-cis-3-methylfentanyl (Burke et al. 1986). This compound depleted about half of the δ-opioid receptors from NG108-15 neuroblastoma × glioma cells at 1 nM concentration. We tritiated this compound to ultra-high specific activity and utilized it to purify the δ-opioid receptor to homogeneity (Simonds et al. 1985). This work allowed researchers to isolate the pure δ-opioid receptor 7 years prior to its availability by cloning.

A later program involved the development of nonpeptide, systemically active δ-selective opioid ligands. We exploited the discovery of BW373U86

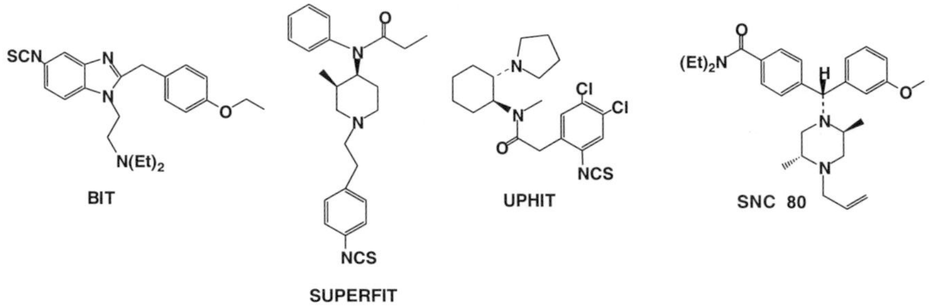

Fig. 14. Structures of affinity labels BIT, SUPERFIT, and UPHIT that label μ-, δ-, and κ-opioid receptors, respectively. Structure of SNC 80, a systemically active δ-opioid receptor agonist.

(a racemate) by Robert McNutt, then at Burroughs-Wellcome Laboratories. This drug contained a novel carbon-nitrogen skeleton and showed δ-mediated effects with some μ-opioid activity. Our first approach was to examine the effect of stereochemistry on selectivity in this series. One of the most interesting compounds to emerge from our initial studies was SNC 80 (Fig. 14), which showed 2000-fold selectivity for the δ- (vs. μ-) opioid receptor (Calderon et al. 1994, 1997) in binding and bioassays. We later showed that SNC 80 was a systemically active δ-opioid receptor agonist with low toxicity in monkeys (Brandt et al. 2001). SNC 80 and related compounds have proven to be valuable research tools for study of the δ-opioid receptor system. We are now developing later-generation compounds in this series and studying those that show higher selectivity in various primate assays.

CONFORMATIONALLY RESTRAINED 5-PHENYLMORPHANS AS OPIOID RECEPTOR PROBES

The 5-phenylmorphans conceptualized and introduced by May in the 1950s are, like the 6,7-benzomorphans, an interesting class of compounds from a practical and theoretical point of view. In the morphine series and in related morphinan-based drugs, only the enantiomer with the absolute stereochemistry (Fig. 9) shown for natural (−)-morphine (5*R*,6*S*,9*R*,13*S*,14*R* absolute configuration) shows significant opioid activity in vivo or in vitro (Jacquet et al. 1977). That is, the unnatural mirror image forms of these compounds *do not* exhibit the well-known effects of natural morphine.

However, in the *N*-methyl-5-(3-hydroxyphenyl)morphans, both enantiomers (Fig. 15) show different and divergent activity (Awaya et al. 1984). The (+)-isomer displays a morphine-like profile, supports morphine dependence in monkeys, and is slightly more potent than morphine as an analgesic in mice. The (–)-isomer, in contrast, is approximately equipotent with morphine in mice but will not support morphine dependence and has weak antagonist effects in monkeys. These findings led to our present program to study these differences.

Our initial approach was to synthesize and pharmacologically evaluate oxide-bridged conformationally restrained analogues (Yamada et al. 2002) that contained a 3-hydroxy group like the parent molecules (Fig. 15). We thought that this research might provide substantial insight into the conformational and configurational requirements for the different activity profiles seen in the parent series. This study presents a considerable synthetic challenge, but can provide valuable insights into the molecular pharmacology of this series of compounds. The challenge arises because in these compounds the oxygen bridge can be attached to six positions, designated a–f (Fig. 15), allowing rotation of the phenyl ring through increments of 60°. Because both an ortho and a para (to the oxide bridge) 3-hydroxy derivative are possible for each of six rotational isomers, this study requires synthesis of six ortho and six para derivatives (12 racemates, 24 enantiomers), each containing four rings and two heteroatoms.

We have now synthesized 10 of the 12 racemates and have identified methodology to generate the final two. Initial binding studies with some of the racemates have identified significant opioid receptor affinity, principally for μ-opioid receptors. Optical resolution of some of the oxide-bridged racemates is in progress and will provide new research tools and potentially new drugs. We have also examined the structure-activity relationships of the N-substituent in the parent (unbridged) series and will apply some of these results in the oxide-bridged series.

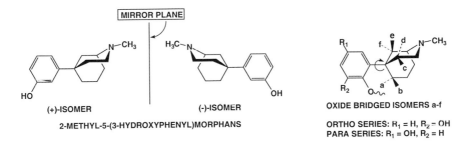

Fig. 15. The enantiomers of 2-methyl-5-(3-hydroxyphenyl)morphan and the general structure of oxide-bridged phenylmorphan isomers a–f. This structure represents 12 monophenolic racemates and 24 enantiomers.

THE FIRST PET IMAGES OF PRIMATE OPIOID RECEPTOR OCCUPANCY

The development of positron emission tomography (PET) as a technique for real time measurement of biochemical function in the brain of human subjects was evolving somewhat parallel to our understanding of the opioid receptor–endorphin system. We and others began programs to develop imaging agents for the opioid receptors. One of our approaches employed a fluorinated derivative of the opioid antagonist naltrexone that became known as (–)-cyclofoxy [(–)-6-β-fluoro-6-desoxynaltrexone] (Burke et al. 1985; Fig. 16). The unlabeled compound showed high-affinity binding in brain homogenates, extensive localization in opioid-receptor-rich regions of rat brain in ex vivo autoradiographic studies, and high potency as an opioid antagonist in animal studies. We labeled the compound with the positron emitting isotope ^{18}F and in December 1984 we published the first PET images of opioid receptor occupancy in the primate brain (Pert et al. 1984).

In the scans, we observed a robust accumulation of [^{18}F](–)-cyclofoxy in the thalamus and caudate nucleus, previously known to be densely populated with opioid receptors from independent studies. The accumulation could be displaced or prevented with therapeutic doses of (–)-naloxone but not by the pharmacologically inert (+)-naloxone prepared by the NIH opiate total synthesis or from (–)-sinomenine. We later synthesized (+)-cyclofoxy (Fig. 16) with the unnatural opiate absolute configuration by the NIH total synthesis. We showed that this variant was pharmacologically inert like (+)-naloxone, and labeled it with ^{18}F. The [^{18}F]labeled (+)-cyclofoxy played a very important role in our PET studies because it did not bind to opioid receptors, but showed nonspecific binding and transport to the brain identical to that of the (–)-isomer. This measurement of nonspecific binding was in excellent agreement with that determined independently in experiments

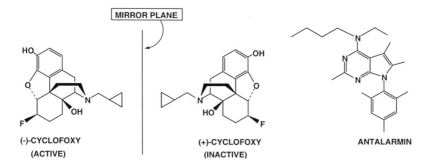

Fig. 16. The enantiomers of cyclofoxy and the corticotropin hormone receptor type 1 antagonist antalarmin.

with [^{18}F](–)-cyclofoxy in which we had saturated the opioid receptors with (–)-naloxone and then directly measured the residual nonspecific binding. In further PET studies, under rigorously demonstrated equilibrium binding conditions with precise measurement of nonspecific binding, we then utilized in vivo Scatchard analysis to quantitate opioid receptor affinity and density in different brain regions in living primates.

Since that time, cyclofoxy has been utilized as a tool for numerous studies in animals and humans that have provided substantial insight into the opioid receptor–endorphin system. It was the first PET ligand to be designed de novo, synthesized, and developed through rodent and primate assays to human PET studies at a single institution. Most recently, a study of former heroin addicts maintained on methadone and normal volunteers revealed 19–32% lower binding of [^{18}F]cyclofoxy (measured relative to the cerebellum) in the methadone-maintained subjects. This finding suggests that occupancy of opioid receptors by methadone was substantial, but that a significant number of unoccupied receptors remained available for normal function (Kling et al. 2000).

CORTICOTROPIN-RELEASING HORMONE RECEPTOR ANTAGONISTS AS MEDICATIONS AND IMAGING AGENTS

A new program in our laboratory focuses on corticotropin-releasing hormone (CRH) and its potential for the study and treatment of drug abuse. This hormone, found in the brain and periphery, is known to be intimately involved in the human response to stress associated with drug abuse (Sarnyai et al. 2001) and in numerous other disorders, including anxiety and depression. In fact, it is involved in virtually all behavioral and physiological components of successful primate adaptation to stressful circumstances (Gilligan et al. 2000). The hormone functions through interaction with well-characterized CRH receptors in the CNS and periphery and subsequent activation of the hypothalamic-pituitary-adrenal axis.

We initiated a program for the design and synthesis of PET and single photon emission computed tomography (SPECT) imaging agents and other drugs for study of this system using CRH antagonist templates from recent patent disclosures by several pharmaceutical companies. Our primary goals in this program are to enable clinical studies of these antagonists in disorders linked to dysfunction of the CRH system and to identify imaging agents for quantitation of CRH receptors in patients with these disorders and in normal human subjects. The combination of clinical studies with receptor quantitation will provide insight into the fundamental nature of drug action and the effects of drug abuse on the CNS, as well as a methodology for the development of clinical correlates with drug receptor dysfunction as adjuncts for diagnoses. This work should provide the ability to further evaluate the effects of treatment on drug abuse and other disorders. In addition, CRH-receptor imaging methodology should be of value in the development of novel medications for the treatment of drug abuse and other disorders in humans.

We initially synthesized a number of fluorine- and iodine-containing ligands (Hsin et al. 2000a; Tian et al. 2001) as potential imaging agents. We also synthesized other compounds (Hsin et al. 2002), some of which have similar affinity (Ki 0.9–3.5 nM) to the lead CRH1 antagonist antalarmin (Ki 2.5 nM, Fig. 16) originated at Pfizer (Chen 1994), and we also prepared ^{13}C double-labeled antalarmin for pharmacokinetic studies (Greiner et al. 2002). In addition, we tritiated one of the fluorine-containing compounds to high specific activity (Hsin et al. 2000b). This drug enters the rat brain but appears too lipophilic to function as a PET ligand; current studies are focused on the identification of a less lipophilic candidate.

We recently designed and synthesized the nonpeptide brominated compound MJL-1-109.2 as a promising second-generation candidate for PET imaging of CRH receptors (M.-J. Lee et al., unpublished data). This compound showed low nanomolar affinity for CRH1 receptors in vitro and a lipophilicity appropriate for a PET ligand. When labeled with the positron-emitting isotope ^{76}Br and examined in autoradiographic studies using slide-mounted rat brain sections, this compound showed high specific binding. It accumulated in the known regional distribution of CRH1 receptors, and this accumulation was prevented by competitive peptide inhibitors and unlabeled MJL-1-109.2 (E. Jagoda et al., unpublished data). We are hopeful that this compound or later-generation compounds now being synthesized will prove to be functional ligands for PET imaging of CRH1-receptor occupancy in animals and humans, just as [^{18}F]cyclofoxy has been for opioid receptors.

In a related set of studies, we have identified several interesting characteristics of the high-affinity CRH1 ligand, antalarmin. We have shown that antalarmin suppresses pituitary ACTH release and peripheral inflammation (Webster et al. 1996). In addition, administration of antalarmin to primates attenuates behavioral, neuroendocrine, and autonomic responses to stress (Habib et al. 2000). Antalarmin also strongly suppresses stress-induced stomach ulcer, colonic hypermotility, and mucin depletion in a rat model of peptic ulcer and irritable bowel syndrome (Gabry et al. 2002). Other studies have shown that CRH plays a central role in blastocyte implantation and prevention of maternal embryo rejection in early pregnancy (Makrigiannakis et al. 2001) and that antalarmin blocks CRH-induced hypertension and attenuates adjuvant-induced arthritis in rats (Webster et al. 2002).

In other studies, we developed a practical synthesis of the $5HT_{2A}$ receptor antagonist MDL100,907, its enantiomer, and their 3-phenolic derivatives as precursors for [^{11}C]-labeled PET ligands (Ullrich and Rice 2000). These results enabled us to utilize PET imaging of $5HT_{2A}$ receptors with [^{11}C]MDL100,907 as a surrogate marker to measure the effect of antalarmin in monkeys. We found that 2-week oral administration of antalarmin downregulated $5HT_{2A}$ receptors in brain regions associated with major neuropsychiatric disorders in a similar way to the inhibitory action of clinically used antidepressants. These and other results suggest that antalarmin and related compounds may be of therapeutic value in some of these disorders (Contoreggi et al. 2003, unpublished data). We are hopeful that our planned clinical studies with antalarmin, together with receptor quantitation through PET studies, will provide much insight into disorders of the CRH system. We recently reviewed the potential utility of nonpeptide CRH1-receptor antagonists as medications and as imaging agents (Contoreggi et al. 2003).

THE CURRENT LABORATORY OF MEDICINAL CHEMISTRY

The permanent staff of the present Laboratory of Medicinal Chemistry, for which I serve as laboratory chief and chief of the Section on Drug Design and Synthesis, includes Wayne Bowen, senior investigator; Wanda Williams, microbiologist; Mariena Mattson, laboratory manager; Paul Kovac, senior investigator, Section on Carbohydrates; and Kathy Ireland-Pardini, secretary. Following Arthur Jacobson's retirement from the NIH in 2001, his successor as biological coordinator for the Drug Evaluation Committee of the CPDD was Andrew Coop (Fig. 7). Coop, a former postdoctoral fellow in the laboratory, is only the fourth biological coordinator since 1930 following Eddy, May, and Jacobson. He is now associate professor in the School of Pharmacy at the University of Maryland, Baltimore.

SUMMARY

This chapter has described some of the major developments in the NIH opiate research program and its predecessor since its inception in 1929. This work began over 70 years ago and has continued at NIH to the present to yield many advances in the fundamental understanding of the chemistry and pharmacology of the opioids and the opioid receptor-endorphin system. More than 750 research papers and patents have resulted from the NIH opiate program. I believe that the following quotation by William C. White applies as much to the NIH analgesic research program as it did to the work of the NRC Committee on Drug Addiction in 1941:

> In the course of man's work many things are begun and some are finished. But work which entails fundamental research is never ended even though an era comes to an end. Those who have participated in the work of the Committee on Drug Addiction of the National Research Council are hopeful that the foundation that has been laid may prove of value not only to contemporary research but to posterity. (White 1941)

ACKNOWLEDGMENTS

Present and former Laboratory of Medicinal Chemistry (LMC) members greatly appreciate support of the LMC program by the National Institute on Diabetes and Digestive and Kidney Diseases and partial support by the National Institute on Drug Abuse. We are also grateful for the long-term contributions of starting materials provided by Mallinckrodt, Inc., which began support of this program in 1934 under Dr. Small's leadership. Lastly, I expresses my sincere appreciation to Dr. Everette L. May for his advice, help, and encouragement during the last 29 years.

REFERENCES

Acker CJ. *Creating the American Junkie: Addiction Research in the Classic Era of Narcotic Control.* Baltimore: Johns Hopkins University Press, 2001.

Archer S, Albertson NF, Harris LS, Pierson AK, Bird JG. Pentazocine: strong analgesics and analgesic antagonists in the benzomorphan series. *J Med Chem* 1964; 7:123–127.

Awaya H, May EL, Aceto MD, et al. Racemic and optically active 2,9-dimethyl-5-(m-hydroxyphenyl)morphans and their pharmacological comparison with the 9-demethyl homologues. *J Med Chem* 1984; 27:536–539.

Brandt MR, Furness MS, Mello NK, Rice KC, Negus SS. Antinociceptive effects of delta-agonists in rhesus monkeys: effects of chemically induced thermal hypersensitivity. *J Pharmacol Exp Ther* 2001; 296:939–946.

Burke TR Jr, Rice KC, Pert CB. Probes for narcotic receptor mediated phenomena. 11. Synthesis of 17-methyl- and 17-cyclopropylmethyl-3,14-dihydroxy-4,5-epoxy-6β-fluoromorphinans (foxy and cyclofoxy) as model opioid ligands suitable for positron emission transaxial tomography. *Heterocycles* 1985; 23:99–106.

Burke TR Jr, Jacobson AE, Rice KC, et al. Probes for narcotic receptor mediated phenomena. 12. Cis-(+)-3-methylfentanylisothiocyanate, a potent site-directed acylating agent for delta opioid receptors: synthesis, absolute configuration and receptor enantioselectivity. *J Med Chem* 1986; 29:1087–1093.

Calderon SN, Rothman RB, Porreca F, et al. Probes for narcotic receptor mediated phenomena. 19. Synthesis of (+)-4-[(αR)-α-(2S,5R)-4-allyl-2,5-dimethyl-1-piperazinyl)-3-methoxybenzyl]-N,N-diethylbenzamide (SNC 80): a highly selective nonpeptide delta receptor agonist. *J Med Chem* 1994; 37:2125-2128.

Calderon SN, Rice KC, Rothman RB, et al. Probes for narcotic receptor mediated phenomena. 23. Synthesis, opioid receptor binding and bioassay of the highly selective delta agonist SNC 80 and related compounds. *J Med Chem* 1997; 40:695–704.

Chen YL. Pyrrolopyrimidines as CRF antagonists. *International Patent Publication* 94/13,676, June 23, 1994.

Contoreggi C, Ayala A, Grant S, et al. Nonpeptide corticotropin releasing hormone type 1 receptor antagonists as medications and imaging agents. *Drugs Future* 2003; 27:1093–1100.

de Costa BR, Band L, Rothman RB, et al. Synthesis of an affinity ligand ('UPHIT') for in vivo acylation of the κ-opioid receptor. *FEBS Lett* 1989; 249:178–182.

Devane WA, Dysarz FA III, Johnson MR, Melvin LS, Howlett AC. Determination and characterization of a cannabinoid receptor in rat brain. *Mol Pharm* 1988; 34:605–613.

Eddy NB. *The National Research Council Involvement in the Opiate Problem 1928–1971*. Washington, DC: National Academy of Sciences, 1973.

Gabry KE, Chrousos GP, Rice KC, et al. Marked suppression of gastric ulcer and intestinal response to stress by a novel class of drugs. *Mol Psychiatry* 2002; 7:474–483.

Gates M, Tschudi G. The synthesis of morphine. *J Am Chem Soc* 1952; 74:1109–1110.

Gates M, Tschudi G. The synthesis of morphine. *J Am Chem Soc* 1956; 78:1380–1393.

Gilligan PJ, Robertson DW, Zaczek R. Corticotropin releasing factor (CRF) receptor modulators; progress and opportunities for new therapeutic agents. *J Med Chem* 2000; 43:1641–1660.

Greiner E, Atkinson AJ, Ayala A, et al. Synthesis of double ^{13}C-labeled antalarmin isotopes for pharmacokinetic studies. *J Labeled Comp Radiopharm* 2002; 45:637–645.

Gulland JM, Robinson R. Constitution of codeine and thebaine. *Mem Proc Manchester Literary Phil Soc* 1925; 69:79–86; *Chem Abstr* 1926; 20:765.

Habib KE, Weld KP, Rice KC, et al. Oral administration of a CRH receptor antagonist significantly attenuates behavioral, neuroendocrine, and autonomic responses to stress in primates. *Proc Natl Acad Sci USA* 2000; 97:6079–6084.

Herkenham M, Lynn AB, Little MD, et al. Cannabinoid receptor localization in brain. *Proc Natl Acad Sci USA* 1990; 87:1932–1936.

Holmes HL. The morphine alkaloids. I and II. In: Manske, RHF, Holmes, HL (Eds). *The Alkaloids*, Vol. 2. New York: Academic Press, 1952, pp 1–216.

Hsin L-W, Webster EL, Chrousos GP, et al. Synthesis and biological activity of fluoro-substituted pyrrolo[2,3-d]pyrimidines: the development of potential positron emission tomography imaging agents for the corticotropin-releasing hormone type-1 receptor. *Bioorg Med Chem Lett* 2000a; 10:707–710.

Hsin L-W, Webster EL, Chrousos GP, et al. Synthesis of [^{3}H](4-fluorobutyl)propyl[2,5,6-trimethyl-7-(2,4,6-trimethylphenyl)pyrrolo[2,3-d]pyrimidin-4-yl]amine: a potent radioligand for corticotropin-releasing hormone type 1 receptor. *J Labeled Comp Radiopharm* 2000b; 43:899–908.

Hsin L-W, Tian X, Webster EL, et al. CRHR$_1$ receptor binding and lipophilicity of pyrrolopyrimidines, potential nonpeptide corticotropin-releasing hormone type 1 receptor antagonists. *Bioorg Med Chem* 2002; 10:175–183.

Iijima I, Rice KC, Silverton JV. Studies in the (+)-morphinan series I. An alternate conversion of (+)-dihydrocodeinone into (+)-codeine. *Heterocycles* 1977; 6:1157–1165.

Iijima I, Minamikawa J-I, Jacobson AE, et al. Studies in the (+)-morphinan series. V. Synthesis and biological properties of (+)-naloxone. *J Med Chem* 1978; 21:398–400.

Jacobson AE, Rice KC. The continuing interrelationship of CPDD and NIDDK. In: Harris LS (Ed). *Problems of Drug Dependence, 1991*. NIDA Research Monograph 119. Washington, DC, 1992, pp 49–53.

Jacquet YF, Klee W, Rice K, Iijima I, Minamikawa J-I. Stereospecific and nonstereospecific effects of (+)-and (–)-morphine: evidence for a new class of receptors? *Science* 1977; 198:842–845.

Johnson MR, Milne GW. *Analgesics*. In: Wolff ME (Ed). *Burger's Medicinal Chemistry*, 4th ed., Part 3. Wiley, 1981, pp 746–747.

Kling MA, Carson RE, Borg L, et al. Opioid receptor imaging with PET and [^{18}F]cyclofoxy in long-term methadone treated former heroin addicts. *J Pharmacol Exp Ther* 2000; 295:1070–1076.

Krueger H, Eddy NB, Sumwalt M. *The Pharmacology of the Opium Alkaloids,* Part 1. Supplement No. 165 to the Public Health Reports. U.S. Government Printing Office, 1941.

Krueger H, Eddy NB, Sumwalt M. *The Pharmacology of the Opium Alkaloids,* Part 2. Supplement No. 165 to the Public Health Reports. U.S. Government Printing Office, 1943.

Makrigiannakis A, Zoumakis E, Kalantariodou S, et al. Corticotropin-releasing hormone promotes blastocyte implantation and early maternal tolerance. *Nature Immunol* 2001; 2:1018–1024.

Matsuda LA, Lolait SJ, Brownstein MJ, Young AC, Bonner TI. Structure of a cannabinoid receptor and functional expression of the cloned cDNA. *Nature* 1990; 346:561–564.

May EL. Dibenzisoquinoline and napthisoquinoline isoquinolino alcohols derived from napthalene. University of Virginia: PhD Dissertation, 1939, pp 1–84.

May EL. Reminiscences and musings of a classical medicinal chemist. *J Med Chem* 1980; 23:225–232.

May EL. The Committee on Problems of Drug Dependence—past, present and future. In: Harris LS (Ed). *Problems of Drug Dependence, 1981.* NIDA Research Monograph 41. Washington, DC, 1982, pp 3–9.

May EL. A half century in medicinal chemistry with major emphasis on pain-relieving drugs and their antagonists. *J Med Chem* 1992; 35:3587–3594.

May EL, Eddy NB. *Synthetic Analgesics Part IIB: 6,7-Benzomorphans,* International Series of Monographs in Organic Chemistry. Oxford: Pergamon, 1969, pp 113–182.

May EL, Jacobson AE. The Committee on Problems of Drug Dependence—a legacy of the National Academy of Sciences: a historical account. *Drug Alcohol Depend* 1989; 23:183–218.

Mosettig E. Lyndon Frederick Small. *Biographical Memoirs of the National Academy of Sciences, USA* 1959:396–413.

Newman AH, Rice KC, Jacobson AE. Potent analgesia, respiratory depression, dependence, abuse liability—clue to separability. In: Harris LS (Ed). *Problems of Drug Dependence, 1991.* NIDA Research Monograph 119. Washington, DC, 1992, pp 54–58.

Palmer DC, Strauss MJ. Benzomorphans: synthesis, stereochemistry, reactions, and spectroscopic characterizations. *Chem Rev* 1977; 77:1–36.

Pert CB, Danks JA, Channing MA, et al. [^{18}F]-3-Acetylcyclofoxy: a useful probe for visualization of opiate receptors in living animals. *FEBS Lett* 1984; 177:281–286.

Rice KC. Synthetic opium alkaloids and derivatives: a short total synthesis of (±)-dihydrothebainone, (±)-dihydrocodeinone, and (±)-nordihydrocodeinone as an approach to a practical synthesis of morphine, codeine, and congeners. *J Org Chem* 1980; 45:3135–3137.

Rice KC. *Short Total Synthesis of Dihydrothebainone, Dihydrocodeinone and Nordihydrocodeinone.* U.S. Patent 4,368,326 issued January 11, 1983.

Rice KC. The development of a practical total synthesis of natural and unnatural codeine, morphine and thebaine. In: Phillipson JD, Roberts MF, Zenk MH (Eds). *The Chemistry and Biology of Isoquinoline Alkaloids.* Berlin: Springer-Verlag, 1985a, pp 191–203.

Rice KC. *A Practical Total Synthesis of Unnatural Enantiomers of Opium-Derived Morphinans.* U.S. Patent 4,521,601 issued June 4, 1985b.

Rice KC. A *Short Total Synthesis of Morphinan Compounds Which Uses Cyclization of a Cycloalkylcarbonyl Compound Selected from Cyclopropylcarbonyl and Cyclobutylcarbonyl.* U.S. Patent 4,613,668, issued September 23, 1986.

Rice KC. Medicinal chemistry in the study of addictive diseases. In: Harris LS (Ed). *Problems of Drug Dependence, 2001.* NIDA Research Monograph 182. Washington, DC, 2002, pp 3–11.

Rice KC, Brossi A. Expedient synthesis of racemic and optically active N-norreticuline, 6'-bromo- and N-substituted N-norreticulines. *J Org Chem* 1980; 45:592–601.

Rice KC, Newman AH. *Total Synthesis of Northebaine, Normorphine and Noroxymorphone Enantiomers and Derivatives via N-Nor Intermediates.* U.S. Patent 5,668,285, issued September 16, 1997.

Rice KC, Ripka WC, Reden J, Brossi A. Pavinan and isopavinan alkaloids: synthesis of racemic and natural thalidine, bisnorargemonine and congeners from N-norreticuline. *J Org Chem* 1980; 45:601–607.

Rice KC, Jacobson AE, Burke TR Jr, et al. Irreversible ligands with high selectivity toward delta or mu opiate receptor subtypes. *Science* 1983; 220:314–316.

Sarnyai Z, Shaham Y, Heinrichs SC. The role of corticotropin-releasing factor in drug addiction. *Pharmacol Rev* 2001; 53:209–243.

Schmidhammer H, Jacobson AE, Brossi A. Chemical and biological study of aromatic oxygenated 6-ketomorphinans. *Med Res Rev* 1983; 3:1–19.

Schwartz MA. *Prescription Drugs in Short Supply: Case Histories.* New York: Marcel Dekker, 1980, pp 9–48.

Simonds WF, Burke TR Jr, Rice KC, Jacobson AE, Klee WA. Purification of the opiate receptor of NG108-15 neuroblastoma x glioma hybrid cells. *Proc Natl Acad Sci USA* 1985; 82:4974–4978.

Small LF. *Chemistry of the Opium Alkaloids.* Supplement No. 103 to the Public Health Reports. U.S. Government Printing Office, 1932.

Small LF, Fitch HM, Smith WE. The addition of organomagnesium halides to pseudocodeine types. II. Preparation of nuclear alkylated morphine derivatives. *J Am Chem Soc* 1936; 58:1457–1463.

Small LF, Eddy NB, Mosettig E, Himmelsbach CK. *Studies on Drug Addiction.* Supplement No. 138 to the Public Health Reports. U.S. Government Printing Office, 1938.

Tian X, Hsin LW, Webster EL, et al. The development of a potential single photon emission computed tomography (SPECT) imaging agent for the corticotropin-releasing hormone receptor type I. *Bioorg Med Chem Lett* 2001; 11:331–333.

Ullrich T, Rice KC. A practical synthesis of the serotonin 5-HT$_{2A}$ receptor antagonist MDL 100907, its enantiomer, and their 3-phenolic derivatives as precursors for [^{11}C]labeled PET ligands. *Bioorg Med Chem* 2000; 8:2427–2432.

Webster EL, Lewis DB, Torpy DJ, et al. *In vivo* and *in vitro* characterization of antalarmin, a novel non-peptide corticotropin-releasing hormone (CRH) receptor antagonist: Suppression of pituitary ACTH release and peripheral inflammation. *Endocrinology* 1996; 137:5747–5750.

Webster EL, Barrientos RM, Contoreggi C, et al. Corticotropin-releasing hormone (CRH) antagonist attenuates adjuvant induced arthritis: evidence supporting a major role for CRH in peripheral inflammation. *J Rheumatol* 2002; 29:1252–1261.

Wilson RS, May EL. 9-Nor-9-hydroxyhexahydrocannabinols, synthesis, some behavioral and analgesic properties, and comparison with the tetrahydrocannabinols. *J Med Chem* 1976; 19:1165–1167.

White WC. *Report of the Committee on Drug Addiction, 1929–1941.* National Research Council, 1941.

Yamada K, Flippen-Anderson JL, Jacobson AE, Rice KC. Probes for narcotic receptor mediated phenomena. 29. Synthesis of rel-(4R,6aR,11bR)-2,3,4,5,6,6a-hexahydro-3-methyl-1*H*-4,11b-methanobenzofuro[3,2-d]azocine-10-ol, the para-a oxide-bridged phenylmorphan isomer, and a new route to rel-(4R,6aR,11bR)-2,3,4,5,6,6a-hexahydro-3-methyl-1*H*-4,11b-methanobenzofuro[3,2-d]azocine-8-ol, the ortho-a oxide-bridged phenylmorphan isomer. *Synthesis* 2002; 16:2359–2364.

Correspondence to: Kenner C. Rice, PhD, Laboratory of Medicinal Chemistry, National Institute of Diabetes and Digestive and Kidney Diseases, National Institutes of Health, Department of Health and Human Services, Bethesda, MD 20892, USA. Tel: 301-496-1856; Fax: 301-402-0589; email: kr21f@nih.gov.

Opioids and Pain Relief: A Historical Perspective,
Progress in Pain Research and Management, Vol.
25, edited by Marcia L. Meldrum, IASP Press,
Seattle, © 2003.

6

The Rise and Demise of the Brompton Cocktail

David Clark

Trent Palliative Care Centre,
University of Sheffield, Sheffield, United Kingdom

The pain field and the modern hospice movement have intertwined histories that we can trace back at least to the early 1950s. In England in 1951, the young social worker Cicely Saunders was urged by a surgeon colleague to study medicine: "It's the doctors who desert the dying and there's so much more to be learned about pain" (Saunders 2000). Just 2 years later, from his base in Seattle, Washington, John Bonica (1953) would publish his ground-breaking treatise on the management of pain. In her pursuit of understanding of the pain of the dying, Saunders, regarded by many as the founder of the modern hospice movement, was soon to turn to the work of Bonica and others in the United States.

On both sides of the Atlantic, problems in recognizing this work arose due to deep skepticism in some quarters and misperceptions about the problem of pain—particularly as it related to chronic conditions and to life-threatening diseases such as cancer. Seen as an inevitable part of the cancer experience, pain was viewed fatalistically by physicians and patients alike. Pain management had for long been the preserve of patent remedies and quackery. Since at least the beginning of the 20th century, the strong narcotics that appeared capable of relieving cancer pain had been viewed with suspicion, and there were concerns, even for patients close to death, about the possibilities of addiction. After World War II, some of these attitudes began to change. A small number of physicians and researchers reconstructed pain as a multifaceted clinical problem that required a combination of strategies for its relief. Pharmacological approaches to pain management became more sophisticated, and so too did the understanding of pain as perception and experience.

The short history of the so-called Brompton cocktail provides some insight into these developments: a pain-relieving elixir that was championed by hospice innovators in Britain, quickly taken up in many parts of the world, and then quite swiftly abandoned in the face of research evidence that questioned its efficacy and brought about its demise. This chapter identifies the clinical purposes that supported the Brompton cocktail and outlines how these came to be served by other approaches within the emerging hospice armamentarium. It also shows how a particular technology of care was disaggregated into a set of clinical, pharmacological, and practical problems through a series of studies conducted by one of the first research programs in modern palliative medicine.

ORIGINS OF THE MIXTURE

Saunders praised the "Brompton mixture" in her first paper, written while she was a medical student and published in 1958. She described the ingredients as nepenthe or liquor of morphine hydrochloride, cocaine hydrochloride, tincture of cannabis, gin, syrup and chloroform water. Her source for the recipe was Richardson and Baker (1956). Such mixtures may be traced at least to the English use of laudanum (opium dissolved in alcohol) in the 18th century. In the 19th century, they flourished in many countries as patent remedies that were freely available. The exact ingredients were always a closely guarded secret, but many, if not most, were based on alcohol, opiates, or both (see Acker, this volume). By the early 20th century, medical reformers had successfully pressed for legislation mandating that contents be described on the label and that certain preparations, notably the opiates, be made available only by medical prescription.

By the time that Saunders offered her support of the Brompton mixture in the late 1950s, several such concoctions for dying patients were already in widespread use in English hospitals. Sir Heneage Ogilvie, consultant surgeon at Guy's Hospital, London, in these years, is an excellent source on the particular virtues of the Brompton mixture, that "great standby in the last days of life." He reports its use and effects thus:

> This mixture is given three times a day. The morphine may be increased to the amount necessary to alleviate pain. The cocaine may also be increased as tolerance is established. Patients taking this mixture rarely need hypodermic injections in addition. The cocaine not merely counteracts the depression occasioned by the morphine, but also gives that wonderful feeling of well-being and exhilaration which makes it the most dangerous

of all the habit-forming drugs. It brings optimism when there is no hope, a certainty of recovery while death comes nearer. (Ogilvie 1957)

The *particular* combination of morphia and cocaine found in the mixture has been traced back by several observers to the work in the late 19th century of Herbert Snow, Surgeon to the Cancer Hospital (later the Royal Marsden), situated in the Brompton neighborhood of London (see Holmes, this volume, for details). Among his various writings, two pamphlets published in 1890 (Snow 1890a,b) are important: *On The Re-appearance (Recurrence) of Cancer after Apparent Extirpation ...* and *The Palliative Treatment of Incurable Cancer, with an Appendix on the Use of the Opium Pipe*. In a paper published in the *British Medical Journal* in September 1896, he enlarged on this latter topic, asserting that malignant disease had its causation in neurosis and arguing that morphia and cocaine, when used in combination, could arrest the progression of the disease and produce "conspicuous improvement, sometimes to a marvellous degree" (Snow 1896). Less than a year later, however, in a letter to the same journal Snow complained that "for imperative reasons of hospital finance I have been reluctantly compelled to abandon this costly medicine [cocaine] for the majority of my hospital patients" (Snow 1897).

It appears that Snow's ideas about combining morphine and cocaine crossed the road (Cale Street) from the Cancer Hospital to the Brompton Hospital. The therapeutic goal of his successors was significantly different, however. For Snow, the chief virtue of the combination was its apparent effect on the progression of cancerous disease, and he seems to have reserved the use of the opium pipe as the chief method for "palliation" and symptom relief in advanced cancer. When the combination was first reported at the Brompton in the early 20th century, its use was recommended for the relief of physical suffering and pain associated with tuberculosis. One writer has suggested that it was Brompton surgeons in the 1920s, such as Arthur Tudor-Edwards and J.E.H. Roberts, who combined morphine and cocaine for oral administration to their post-thoracotomy lung cancer patients (Kerrane 1975), making the mixture palatable with a syrup base of gin and honey. Its development has also been attributed to the chest physician Clifford Hoyle at King's College Hospital, London, in the 1930s (Hinton 1996), who was certainly writing about its use from at least the late 1940s (Hoyle 1948). Saunders (1993) records that by 1935, the Brompton mixture was in use as part of a regimen of "regular giving" of pain relief at St. Luke's Hospital, Bayswater, one of a small number of homes for the dying founded in London at the end of the 19th century.

By mid-century, such cocktails had been widely adopted in English hospitals and were prescribed for the terminal patient, both on demand and at regular intervals. In 1952, when the Brompton Hospital produced its own supplement to the *National Formulary*, the mixture appeared in print for the first time, under the name *Haustus E.* (*Haustus* meaning a draught or potion, and *E.* perhaps *euphoriens*; Hinton 1996). This version was listed in Martindale's *Extra Pharmacopoeia* in 1958. In 1976 it finally appeared in the *British National Formulary*. By then, it had gradually come to be known by several different names: Brompton cocktail, Brompton mixture, *Mistura euphoriens, Mistura pro moribunda, Mistura pro euthanasia,* Saunders' mixture, and Hoyle's mixture. Indeed, when the first modern hospices opened in the United Kingdom, they too adopted their own nomenclatures, as at St. Luke's Hospice, Sheffield, where there were several variants: St. Luke's mild, St. Luke's moderate, followed (rather coyly) by St. Luke's "individual" (B. Noble, personal communication, 2001).

As the use of the mixture spread, its contents varied among institutions. The alcohol could take the form of gin, whisky, or brandy and could be added in various quantities according to patient preference. A phenothiazine was often added, either prochlorperazine or chlorpromazine, for both antiemetic and sedative purposes. Evidence suggests that in France, an antihistamine such as promethazine was also being included in similar mixtures called "lytic cocktails" (Meunier-Cartal et al. 1995). Most significantly, some practitioners in the United Kingdom favored diamorphine (diacetylmorphine, heroin) over morphine because of its apparently more rapid action; some even dropped the cocaine and instead used morphine and diamorphine together in the mixture (Anonymous 1979).

Even in the late 1950s and early 1960s, the use of such cocktails was not viewed unproblematically. First, there was the question of the mixture's purpose. The Brompton cocktail was associated historically with covert euthanasia. John Hinton, a pioneer of early research on the care of the dying in the United Kingdom in the 1960s, recalled in 1996:

> [W]as it in fact hastening people's death, rather than just being an analgesic and euphoriant as they thought at that point? ... and they said, "Well there was nothing we could do, let's start him off on the cocktail." And sometimes it was very appropriate because the person was in pain ... there was nothing you could do. Sometimes it was a bit inappropriate; that they were only just beginning to feel a bit of discomfort, and nowadays it would have been managed differently by grading the analgesics. And sometimes one had the feeling it was used to, at least, tidy things up a bit, at least in people's minds, and this is where all the misgivings arose. And one would

… go round doing a night round and a night nurse would say, "Well, they've just started him off on the cocktail and I don't think it's right because he's not ready for it yet." … And you sometimes wondered about the motivation.

Nonclinical motives were also attributed for use of the mixture. A well-cited (and probably apocryphal) example is that of King George V's doctor, Lord Dawson of Penn, who may have administered the Brompton cocktail to ensure the time of the King's death so that the first obituary would appear in *The Times*, rather than a less appropriate newspaper.

Another question was the real efficacy of the mixture in relieving pain, particularly because there were doubts about the potency of narcotics when taken by mouth, rather than injection. Saunders reported, however, that the mixture "may be adequate" for the relief of severe pain (Saunders 1960). Overall, it appears that physicians and nursing staff preferred the cocktail for several reasons. It relieved the patient of the necessity for regular and painful injections and could be made available at home as well as in the hospital. Likewise, it could be placed by the bed for patients to take as required, and was easily administered during the night. The Brompton cocktail might be described as "patient-friendly"; it was a means of reducing dependence upon the doctor, the nurse, and the hypodermic.

The alcoholic vehicle also seems to have appealed to some patients, although not to others; the idea of using specific alcoholic beverages, rather than ethyl alcohol only, seems to have been associated with the notion of patients making personal choices about their therapy (Culver-James 1979). Among patients in London's East End, cared for at St. Joseph's Hospice, the cocktail was apparently very acceptable. Varying the gin (a popular working-class drink in London from Victorian times) with brandy seems to have been a way of making the elixir more personal; it was made up at the bedside, according to preference. Other, more unusual, beverages could be used, such as "crème de menthe for a patient who is liable to indigestion" (Ogilvie 1957).

In English hospitals of the 1950s and early 1960s, variations on the Brompton mixture seem to have been primarily associated with the care of patients suffering from pain near the end of life. It was Saunders' work in promoting the mixture through her writings, and her strong influence on other hospice founders, that helped to establish it as a key "technology" in the emerging work of the modern hospice movement as well. Precisely because she was also interested in research on pain and pain relief, however, the mixture came under scrutiny in an early program of work conducted at her model facility, St. Christopher's Hospice, which opened in south London in 1967.

SCRUTINIZING THE COCKTAIL

Robert Twycross was still an undergraduate student in 1963 when he first met Cicely Saunders after attending a lecture she gave in Bristol. The following year, he created the Radcliffe Christian Medical Society simply in order to give a pretext for inviting her to speak in Oxford. They formed a rapport, and after he qualified as a physician, she began to encourage him to think about full-time work in what was then being called "terminal care" (Twycross 1996). So it was that in 1968 an invitation came to join her team at St. Christopher's, where she was eager to embark upon a program of research in palliative care. She had asked Colin Murray Parkes to conduct a series of studies to compare the quality of service at the hospice to that given in local hospitals. Saunders hoped that Twycross would conduct basic studies of the pain relief methods she had developed during her years at St. Joseph's Hospice, methods based on her clinical intuition and judgment, which had yet to be tested by the more probing tool of the randomized controlled trial. He declined her first offer, however, in favor of completing his MRCP; only in 1971 did he finally arrive at St. Christopher's as a clinical research fellow. The pharmacologist Duncan Vere agreed to supervise his research. Twycross and Vere opened up the Brompton cocktail to scientific scrutiny for the first time, in a program of studies generated by Saunders' clinical observations. (Some earlier studies had been carried out at St. Christopher's by Ronald Welldon.)

The research, conducted over several years, focused on a number of areas: standardization of the mixture, the relationship between the active constituents and the vehicle, the keeping properties of the mixture, the action of cocaine as part of the cocktail, and the relative efficacy of morphine and diamorphine. Between 1972 and 1979, some 39 publications addressed these questions and other issues of pain relief for the dying patient. Of considerable scientific interest, these publications carried perhaps a greater symbolic importance in offering research support for a novel therapeutic perspective.

Saunders had written persuasively and at length about the benefits of her approach; she had coined the term "total pain" to highlight the multifaceted characteristics of suffering, including physical, social, psychological, and emotional aspects (Clark 1999). She presented a view of chronic pain as a problem of meaning, for such pain can be timeless, endless, meaningless, bringing a sense of isolation and despair. Indeed, it could be experienced as "not just an event, or a series of events ... but rather a situation in which the patient is, as it were, held captive" (Saunders 1970). In terminally ill patients, a major challenge was to avoid the onset of chronic pain by active strategies of prevention. In particular, Saunders advocated the regular giving of strong analgesia in anticipation of, rather than in response to, the onset of pain. This practice generated the oft-repeated Saunders maxim: "constant pain needs constant control." At the same time, she emphasized the value of the caregiver's willingness to listen, citing the words of one patient who said "the pain seemed to go by just talking." In Saunders' work, the pain of terminal illness came to be regarded as an illness in itself. Her use of drugs, particularly strong opiate drugs and the cocktail, was not simply a matter of therapeutic technique, but also the expression of her commitment as physician to her patient. The readily available, "patient-friendly" Brompton mixture symbolized the power and personal nature of that commitment. "Total care" was the therapeutic response to "total pain."

Twycross used the tools of research to test out some of these ideas, to scrutinize the hospice method, and, in particular, to assess the pharmacology of the Brompton cocktail as part of Saunders' therapeutic program. A second line of enquiry concerned the relative benefits of morphine and diamorphine. In a paper written with colleagues from the Epsom Hospital Laboratories, Twycross advanced the case for the *oral* administration of strong narcotics, demonstrating from a study of urinary excretion that "an orally administered solution of diamorphine hydrochloride is completely absorbed by the gastrointestinal tract but … a solution of morphine sulphate is only two-thirds absorbed" (Twycross et al. 1974). The difference, he suggested, could be allowed for in the dosage.

In the same year, Twycross (1974) reported on a survey of 90 teaching and district general hospitals in the United Kingdom that showed marked variation in the composition of "elixirs" for the relief of pain and suffering in terminal cancer. He supported the introduction of a standard diamorphine and cocaine mixture in the *British Pharmaceutical Codex,* but raised questions about its keeping properties. Another issue addressed in this paper concerned the broad acceptability of a mixture that some patients experienced as either extremely nauseating or unacceptably alcoholic. Interestingly, the issue of palatability seemed to occupy more attention than possible concerns about addiction. Above all, Twycross emphasized the need to "evaluate objectively the contribution of the cocaine to the pharmacological effect of the mixture" (Twycross 1974).

Across the Atlantic, others had been influenced by the British hospice movement's adoption of the Brompton mixture as well as by Saunders' notion of "total pain." In Canada, Balfour Mount, Ronald Melzack, and colleagues began a series of studies within a newly opened palliative care service in Montreal. Their early findings suggested that "the Brompton mixture provides convenient and uniform pain control without important adverse effects"

(Mount et al. 1976). They reported that the mixture relieved the pain of 90% of patients in the palliative care unit and of 75–80% of those in the general wards and private rooms. The Montreal team concluded that the results were consistent with the gate control theory of pain and that the Brompton mixture "does not act on only a single dimension of pain but has a strong effect on the sensory, affective and evaluative dimensions together" (Melzack et al. 1976). So far, it seemed, the traditional elixir, albeit with a more specifically defined makeup, had survived the transition from old-style care of the dying to the new world of palliative care.

At St. Christopher's, Twycross had decided to assess not only the value of the elixir as a whole, but also the merits of its constituent elements— especially because diamorphine and morphine had become almost interchangeable in the clinical usage of the mixture in England. Two important studies, which had a major impact on subsequent clinical practice, were reported in 1977. The first paper, which appeared in *Pain* (Twycross 1977a), described a comparative trial of diamorphine and morphine, in which the two drugs were administered regularly in a version of the Brompton mixture containing cocaine hydrochloride in a 10-mg dose. A total of 699 patients entered the trial, and 146 of these crossed over after 2 weeks from diamorphine to morphine, or vice versa; the crossover mechanism allowed the researchers to test for the effects of individual variability in response. A previously determined potency ratio of 1.5:1 was used. In the female crossover patients, no difference was noted in relation to pain or other symptoms evaluated, but male crossover patients experienced more pain and were more depressed while receiving diamorphine, which suggests an error in the potency ratio. Twycross concluded that if the relative difference in potency was correctly determined, both oral morphine and oral diamorphine would provide effective pain relief, but that the more soluble diamorphine retained certain advantages in patients requiring injections of high dosages.

In the second trial, reported in a letter to the *British Medical Journal,* the morphine and diamorphine elixirs were compared with and without a 10-mg dose of cocaine (Twycross 1977b). Forty-five patients made satisfactory crossovers; the trends within the morphine and diamorphine groups were similar, and were combined for purposes of analysis. The study showed that patients who crossed over to a cocaine-added mixture after 2 weeks showed a small but statistically significant increase in alertness, but those who changed to a noncocaine mixture showed no detectable change in alertness or pain relief. Twycross concluded that the addition of cocaine, at this standard dosage, was of borderline efficacy.

As a result of his work, the routine use of the combination of cocaine and diamorphine at St. Christopher's was abandoned; instead, morphine was prescribed alone in chloroform water, together with an antiemetic where indicated. As Saunders (2000) put it: "So one day in May 1977 all the patients who were on oral diamorphine went onto oral morphine and the only people who turned a hair were the doctors who had to write out all the drug charts." On May 24, 1977, the very day of the changeover, Saunders wrote to Helen Nowoswiat at the Roswell Park Memorial Institute in Buffalo, New York, that "for teaching purposes we should no longer use a drug [diamorphine] which is unavailable in most of the world" and added: "I do not think there is any need for your physician to conduct a further study in this area" (Clark 2002).

Supporting evidence came 2 years later from the Canadian researchers, who also reported a double-blind crossover comparison of a standard Brompton cocktail containing morphine, cocaine, ethyl alcohol, syrup, and chloroform water with oral morphine alone in a flavored water solution. Pain was measured using the McGill Pain Questionnaire, and the patients, their nurses, and relatives provided ratings of confusion, nausea, and drowsiness. The study showed no significant difference between the cocktail and the oral morphine alone; both relieved pain in about 85% of patients, with no significant differences in detrimental side effects. The Canadians adopted the name "elixir of morphine" for the morphine solution (Melzack et al. 1979).

LINGERING DEMISE OF THE BROMPTON MIXTURE

As one of three papers presented at the First International Symposium on Pain in Advanced Cancer in Venice in 1978, Twycross (1979) drew together his summative statement on the matter. There had been, he suggested, a tendency to "endow the Brompton cocktail with almost mystical properties and to regard it as the panacea for terminal cancer pain." Generously, he allowed that if the physician were aware of the potential side effects of the main ingredients, then its use might be maintained. But set against this were the inconveniences to the pharmacist, the potential unpalatability to the patient, the higher financial costs incurred, and the restricted potential for the physician to manipulate the dosage. Clinical pharmacology had revealed that the Brompton cocktail was no more than a dressed-up way of administering oral morphine to cancer patients in pain. It was about to become part of the mythic prehistory of the new palliative care movement.

Several accounts describe how the Brompton cocktail fell from favor. Tony Crowther, later medical director of St. Luke's Hospice in Sheffield, recalled how he used the cocktail in general practice during the 1970s:

Well, I stopped using it, but not for the reason we don't use it now. I mean we don't use it now because when you double it up for pain control, you double up all the other stuff in it. I actually stopped using it because I got fed up with ordering it, and of course there were two basic recipes: one with gin in it and one with brandy in it. And I always got it wrong, or it seemed that I always got it wrong, and the patient said, "Oh, I don't like gin." So you had to throw this wonderful stuff away and get one with brandy in [laughs] or the other way round. ... [Also] the messages were coming from Cicely Saunders and St. Christopher's that it was wrong to have mixtures. The Department of Health were beginning to say, guide prescribing a little bit, and that mixtures or pills containing two drugs ... had potential danger for doubling up everything, if you increased the dose. So I think it was really a combination of all those things that made us change. (Crowther 1996)

Despite the "official" pronouncements, the Brompton cocktail lived on for a while. Interviews conducted as part of the Hospice History Project at the University of Sheffield suggest that it stayed in use in community services and in some British hospitals during the 1980s. It was occasionally endorsed in the American professional literature (Glover et al. 1980), where it was often referred to as "Brompton's mixture," and was promoted by supporters of a proposed Compassionate Pain Relief Act (which would also have legalized medicinal heroin in the United States) in 1984. A physician in Ibadan, Nigeria, reported its use for cancer pain there to the World Health Organization in 1982 (Swerdlow Papers 1982). The Brompton cocktail had flowered briefly but vividly in the early days of the modern hospice movement, and the influence of the new movement gave it a long half-life. Certainly it stayed in use long after its early promoters first urged its demise.

Saunders' correspondence reveals numerous international inquiries about the cocktail, continuing into at least the mid-1980s. She wrestled with the difficulties of discouraging the use of a therapy she had long championed and promoting instead the regular giving of oral morphine, a drug that also had its detractors. On June 28, 1977, she wrote to Dr. Richard Lamberton at St. Joseph's Hospice, in Hackney, London, where almost 20 years previously she had begun her first systematic attempts to relieve pain using the mixture:

We have a real problem with the Brompton Cocktail. As you no doubt know it is becoming an acceptable form of treatment in the U.S. under that title and with flexible dosage and usually without cocaine. It may be that we have to accept it, putting it in quotes and pointing out that it is by no means the same dose every time, nor was it when it was first concocted at the Brompton as far as I know. Now we have diamorphine elixir in the B.P. we are standardising it but as we are stopping diamorphine anyway that does not really help. Perhaps this should be a topic for the Therapeutics Conference in November. (Clark 2002)

A year later (May 18, 1978), she wrote to an American inquirer, Kathleen Mavrevitch of Rosedale, New York:

> We do not call our mixture by the name of the Brompton Hospital and, as you see, we have simplified it considerably. We have not noticed a difference in the wards as a whole since we both changed the morphine and omitted the cocaine, but this was of course based on controlled clinical trials to back up this clinical impression. ... I have been using a narcotic mixture since 1948 in various settings and am convinced that this is a convenient way of giving strong analgesics—and very acceptable to patients. It is, however, much more the way you use your drugs and your total care of the patient which is of greater importance. (Clark 2002)

Four years later (May 20, 1982) she repeated the same point to Cesar Pantoja of Bogota, Colombia:

> There are many different versions of the "Brompton Mixture" but you will find here in the enclosed reprint the prescription which we are using. Chloroform water is used as being bacteriostatic and as a help with the unpleasant taste of the narcotic. ... If there is no way of making this available in your country you will also see in the reprint a number of alternative narcotic drugs with their equivalent dosage and dose intervals. It is not so much the drug that you use as the way that you use it, although we ourselves find morphine the most flexible, especially when one is balancing the dose to the patient's need. (Clark 2002)

Saunders' argument was that several different drug therapies might both relieve pain and maintain alertness, even over the longer term, but that any drug was most effective when combined with a holistic view of the patient and not a simple diagnosis of physical pain. Within this humanist perspective, it was best to use the drug that was most acceptable, most widely available, and most flexible—morphine. As she wrote to Jean Ihli of Hartford, Connecticut, in 1980:

> You are quite right in that we have carried out work which has shown that we can use morphine as effectively as heroin. We certainly have patients on long term use of morphine who are alert and capable of living in their own homes and so on. In order to completely alleviate pain the patient does not have to be rendered unconscious if each area of pain, such as bone pain, is treated specifically and the patient is seen as a person with his mental, social and spiritual needs. (Clark 2002)

There continued to be those, such as Dr. O'Connell of Penang, who doubted the efficacy of morphine alone by mouth, and Saunders could be heated in her response:

> I really am not going to give up! Diamorphine and morphine when used in equi-analgesic doses, individually titrated to the patient's need, are both excellent analgesics. Robert Twycross's study showed that given regularly by mouth with a phenothiazine, there was no observable clinical difference either physically in the form of side effects or in the emotional state. If you have found it [morphine] a poor analgesic or had to use another analgesic when giving a Brompton mixture then I am sure that you must have been giving an inadequate dose. (Clark 2002)

IMPLICATIONS

It is not difficult to see the fall of the Brompton cocktail as part of a wider sea-change in the science and art of terminal care. We might capture this as a shift from a "traditional" mode of thinking and practice to one that is distinctly modern in character. Potions, mixtures, and above all, elixirs carry ancient associations, reaching back to earlier periods in the history of medical practice. They can be invested with mystical, even alchemical properties, their actions as clouded as their appearance. At the same time, as the varying names of this particular mixture reveal, the purposes of its use were also somewhat ambiguous. Was it intended to induce euphoria? Did it potentiate moribundity? Most intriguing of all, was it originally intended to bring about an "easeful" death or even to hasten death?

There seems to be no doubt that the Brompton cocktail was spoken about euphemistically by doctors and nurses, and that patients and their families were influenced by this language. The idea of a "cocktail" or "elixir" rather than a "drug" suggested that the last days of life might be enjoyed, that a single magic potion might comfort all the miseries of "total pain." Clearly, for Saunders, the message of reassurance that the name of the mixture conveyed to the patient was as significant as its pharmaceutical properties. Such ways of communicating are hard to abandon—witness the McGill term "morphine elixir" for a mixture that contained only the drug itself and water.

An allegedly more rational approach has been adopted to the management of pain since the demise of the Brompton cocktail. Physicians continue to prescribe combinations of drugs for palliative care patients (often for purposes for which they are not licensed); narcotics for pain relief are accompanied by antidepressants, antiemetics, laxatives, and other drugs. But the new and important watchword is *titration*—something much harder to do with the varied ingredients of the cocktail. For a magic mixture, the physician must substitute attention to the individual patient, which is both more demanding and potentially more meaningful.

Encouraged by Saunders and mentored by Vere, Twycross saw the possibility of refracting science through the varied colors of the Brompton cocktail. In current sociological parlance, he "deconstructed" the cocktail and revealed it as several things: a set of pharmacological problems, a practical matter of manufacturing and safe storage, a question of patient preferences, a symbolic element in the culture of terminal care, and above all, a turning point in thinking about and practicing pain control. His work, and that of colleagues from Europe and North America, outlined a new model of pain management, in which opioid drugs could be used safely and with predictable efficacy, and without the need for mystery, magic, or a gin chaser.

ACKNOWLEDGMENTS

Research for this paper was funded by a grant to study "Innovations in cancer pain relief: technologies, ethics and practices," awarded in the United Kingdom as part of the U.K. Economic and Social Research Council/Medical Research Council program on Innovative Health Technologies (grant number L218252055). The author is grateful to the Wellcome Trust (grant numbers 043877/Z/95 and 058078/Z/99) for its support of the work of the Hospice History Project.

REFERENCES

Anonymous. Brompton Cocktail. Editorial. *Lancet* 1979; 9:1220–1221.

Bonica JJ. *The Management of Pain.* Philadelphia: Lea and Febiger, 1953.

Clark D. "Total pain," disciplinary power and the body in the work of Cicely Saunders, 1958–1967. *Soc Sci Med* 1999; 49:727–736.

Clark D. *Cicely Saunders, Founder of the Hospice Movement: Selected Letters, 1959–1999.* Oxford: Oxford University Press, 2002.

Crowther A. Oral History Interview, conducted by Clark D. Sheffield: Hospice History Project Collection, Sheffield Palliative Care Studies Group, University of Sheffield, December 1996.

Culver-James J. The Brompton Mixture. *Can Med Assoc J* 1979; 120:1331.

Glover DD, Lowry TJ, Jacknowitz AI. Brompton's mixture in alleviating pain of terminal neoplastic disease. *South Med J* 1980; 73:278–282.

Hinton J. Oral History Interview, conducted by Clark D. Sheffield: Hospice History Project Collection, Sheffield Palliative Care Studies Group, University of Sheffield, April 1996.

Hoyle C. The care of the dying. In: *Index to Treatment*, 13th ed. Bristol: John Wright and Son, 1948.

Kerrane TA. The Brompton Cocktail. *Nurs Mirror* 1975; May:59.

Melzack R, Ofiesh JG, Mount BM. The Brompton mixture: effects on pain in cancer patients. *Can Med Assoc J* 1976; 115:125–129.

Melzack R, Mount BM, Gordon JM. The Brompton mixture versus morphine solution given orally: effects on pain. *Can Med Assoc J* 1979; 20:435–438.

Meunier-Cartal RN, Souberbielle JC, Boureau F. Morphine and the "Lytic Cocktail" for terminally ill patients in a French general hospital: evidence for an inverse relationship. *J Pain Symptom Manage* 1995; 10:267–273.

Mount BM, Ajemian I, Scott JF. Use of the Brompton mixture in treating the chronic pain of malignant disease. *Can Med Assoc J* 1976; 115:122–124.

Ogilvie H. Journey's end. *Practitioner* 1957; 179:584–591.

Richardson JS, Baker D. The management of terminal disease. In: Richardson JS (Ed). *The Practice of Medicine*. London: Churchill, 1956.

Saunders C. Dying of cancer. *St Thomas's Hospital Gazette* 1958; 56:37–47.

Saunders C. The management of patients in the terminal stage. In: Raven R (Ed). *Cancer,* Vol. 6. London: Butterworth, 1960.

Saunders C. Nature and management of terminal pain. In: Shotter EF (Ed). *Matters of Life and Death*. London: Darton, Longman and Todd, 1970.

Saunders C. Oral History Interview, conducted by Clark D. Sheffield: Hospice History Project Collection, Sheffield Palliative Care Studies Group, University of Sheffield, May 2000.

Saunders C, Doyle D, Hanks G, MacDonald N (Eds). *The Oxford Textbook of Palliative Medicine*. Oxford: Oxford University Press, 1993, pp v–viii.

Snow HL. *The Palliative Treatment of Incurable Cancer: With an Appendix on the Use of the Opium Pipe*. London: Churchill, 1890a.

Snow HL. *On the Re-appearance (Recurrence) of Cancer after Apparent Extirpation, with Suggestions for Its Prevention*. London: Churchill, 1890b.

Snow HL. Opium and cocaine in the treatment of cancerous disease. *BMJ* 1896; September:718–719.

Snow HL. The opium-cocaine treatment of malignant disease. *BMJ* 1897; April:1019.

Swerdlow M (Comp). *Mark Swerdlow Papers,* John C. Liebeskind History of Pain Collection, Louise M. Darling Biomedical Library, University of California, Los Angeles, 1982.

Twycross RG. Diamorphine and cocaine elixir BPC 1973. *Pharm J* 1974; 212:153–159.

Twycross RG. Choice of strong analgesic in terminal cancer: diamorphine or morphine? *Pain* 1977a; 3:93–104.

Twycross RG. Value of cocaine in opiate-containing elixirs. *BMJ* 1977b; 2:1348.

Twycross RG. The Brompton Cocktail. In: Bonica JJ, Ventafridda V (Eds). *International Symposium on Pain of Advanced Cancer,* Advances in Pain Research and Therapy, Vol. 2. New York: Raven Press, 1979, pp 291–300.

Twycross RG. Oral History Interview, conducted by Clark D. Sheffield: Hospice History Project Collection, Sheffield Palliative Care Studies Group, University of Sheffield, January 1996.

Twycross RG, Fry DE, Wills PD. The alimentary absorption of diamorphine and morphine in man as indicated by urinary excretion studies. *Br J Clin Pharmacol* 1974; 1:491–494.

Correspondence to: David Clark, PhD, Institute for Health Research, Alexandra Square, Lancaster University, Lancaster LA1 4YT, United Kingdom.

Opioids and Pain Relief: A Historical Perspective,
Progress in Pain Research and Management, Vol.
25, edited by Marcia L. Meldrum, IASP Press,
Seattle, © 2003.

7

The Dawn of Endorphins

Huda Akil

*Departments of Neuroscience and Psychiatry and Mental Health Research
Institute, University of Michigan, Ann Arbor, Michigan, USA*

This chapter covers a particularly interesting time of convergence for the study of the neurobiology of pain, the emergence of endorphins, and the integration of neuroscience, pharmacology, and behavior. I am a scientist, not a trained historian, so this account will not be complete in covering all aspects of the history. In addition, space limitations prevent me from mentioning all those who have done wonderful work during this era. I will relate my perspective as a spectator and participant, a young researcher who had a lot to learn, but who realized she was witnessing a wonderful moment in the history of science. For readers who want to learn more, let me recommend the *Anatomy of Scientific Discovery* (Goldberg 1988).

The story began in the Liebeskind laboratory in Franz Hall at the University of California Los Angeles (UCLA). When I arrived to begin my doctoral work with John Liebeskind, he was interested in what was called central pain—puzzling phenomena such as phantom limb pain and other pain experiences for which physicians could not find a clear source, injury, or lesion in the periphery. Liebeskind was interested in the brain sites associated with central pain. He based his early research on neurosurgical papers reporting that electrical stimulations of certain sites in the brain prompted patient reports of pain and severe discomfort, and assigning painful sensations to the periphery even without objective evidence of peripheral injury.

This surgically observed phenomenon represented the model that Liebeskind was searching for. His students (Tom Wolfle, David Mayer, and I, and several others who followed) began to lower electrodes into a particular area of animal brains to ascertain whether we could mimic the phenomenon of central pain by electrical stimulation. As the starting point we chose an area termed the periaqueductal gray, which had been identified in the human studies as triggering the phenomenon akin to central pain. Wolfle and Mayer discovered that passing a tiny current in the ventral area of this gray matter profoundly altered the animal's behavior. We were expecting to see increased pain, but instead we saw decreased pain, although when the current was very high, the animal became uncomfortable.

For example, when we placed a rat in a bucket of ice and passed that tiny current, the rat would just sit there as if it was not very cold. Given something to eat, the rat would sit and nibble on it. When we turned the current off, the rat would leap out and behave as if feeling very uncomfortable. While we passed the current into its brain, we could pinch or poke the animal and subject it to slightly or moderately painful stimuli, and it would be unresponsive. The rat did not appear to feel pain, even though alert and awake. We thus called this phenomenon "stimulation-produced analgesia" or SPA. We later learned that Reynolds (1969) had independently observed a similar phenomenon of profound inhibition of pain reactivity (analgesia) with activation of the central gray area. His approach and conditions were sufficiently different from ours, so the convergence of evidence was convincing—the brain appeared to have a powerful mechanism for blocking pain in the periaqueductal gray region.

For his Ph.D. dissertation, Mayer, the senior graduate student, mapped the brain sites that can induce SPA. He discovered an expanse of gray region surrounding the third ventricle, the aqueduct, and even the rostral aspects of the fourth ventricle—termed the periaqueductal and periventricular sites—that could produce analgesia upon electrical stimulation. This realization not only extended the previous findings to beyond the periaqueductal gray, but suggested an extensive and complex system for modulating pain in the core of the brain.

When the time came to publish this work, we looked to the scientific literature to relate the SPA phenomenon to other mechanisms of pain control. One of Mayer's colleagues at UCLA (Bruce Carder) said, "You should look up the work by a Chinese scientist called Tsou. You will find it interesting." Indeed, this paper in a Chinese journal called *Scientia Sinica* (Tsou and Zhang 1964) was most relevant. The authors were searching for the sites of morphine action and reported the first effort to microinject morphine into the brains of rabbits and measure the animals' responsiveness to painful stimuli. They tested sites all over the brain and found that the best place to produce pain relief with morphine was exactly in those core gray regions that we had identified by electrical stimulation as responsible for the inhibition of pain responses.

We thus realized that this powerful way of inhibiting pain might bear a relationship to the anatomical basis for opioid analgesia. We had this idea before anyone had isolated opioid receptors or their ligands, the endorphins.

A paper in *Science* by Mayer and colleagues (1971) proposed that "stimulation attenuates pain by activating a neural substrate that functions normally in the blockage of pain. That such a substrate exists and is capable of being selectively activated was supported by a number of studies concerning the site and mechanism of the analgesic action of morphine."

At the time, our hypothesis met with some disbelief. Around 1970 I remember meeting Jim Olds of the California Institute of Technology. He was an extremely prominent physiological psychologist (Liebeskind had worked with him as a graduate student at the University of Michigan) and one of my scientific heroes, whose work had originally inspired me to move into a more biological area of psychology. Olds had discovered the phenomenon of self-stimulation, whereby an animal works (e.g., presses a lever) to activate electrically certain brain regions that appear to be highly rewarding. We in the Liebeskind group saw SPA as a parallel to self-stimulation, with one neural system blocking pain and the other generating positive reinforcement. Olds, however, seemed skeptical. He told me, "You are probably just jamming up the circuitry of pain transmission. This is most likely not an active process. How do you know it is an active process?" While his skepticism was unsettling, it led us to ask some important questions and in many ways inspired the framing of my dissertation work. The question became: Does SPA truly represent an organized brain mechanism for inhibiting pain, or were our experiments just creating a functional lesion in the normal pain-processing pathways?

We conducted several studies to elucidate the phenomenon. For my doctoral thesis, under Liebeskind's supervision, I attempted to show that this analgesic mechanism was not disruptive, but an active process, in the sense that it depended on neurotransmission. At the time, we knew the most about the monoamine neurotransmitters, so the idea was to use the known antagonists of monoaminergic systems and show that they would interfere with the SPA process. For example, I used blockers for serotonin and norepinephrine, and made the direct analogy between SPA and morphine analgesia. How morphine worked at the level of the brain was already a subject of interest. Cheney and Goldstein and others had shown, for example, that P-chlorophenylalanine (PCPA), a drug that blocks serotonin transmission, also blocks some of the actions of morphine (Cheney and Goldstein 1971). My thesis work showed a similar effect on SPA, and used the parallels between morphine analgesia and SPA to prove that the latter phenomenon was a neurally organized process, and not merely a nonspecific lesion of the brain (Akil and Mayer 1972).

In carrying this idea to its extreme, we became interested in characterizing the SPA phenomenon as if it were morphine. We wanted to see if it produced tolerance and dependence, and whether SPA could be blocked by opiate antagonists. I began to read the opiate literature and discovered a commonly used drug called nalorphine, which was a mixed agonist-antagonist. I tried to give nalorphine immediately prior to SPA, but found that nalorphine in itself was an agonist that could inhibit pain responsiveness. After waiting for the nalorphine analgesia to wear off, I would stimulate the animal and show that it was less analgesic than under no-drug or predrug conditions. Given the complex nature of nalorphine, this experiment was not perfect, but it suggested that opiate antagonists might block the endogenous pain-modulating system.

As a graduate student, I remember attending a meeting (the 1971 Winter Conference on Brain Research) with E. Leong Way, the chair of pharmacology at the University of California San Francisco, and telling him about these results. "Nalorphine is a dirty drug; use naloxone," he suggested. I had never heard of naloxone, but I obtained a sufficient quantity and tried it in the context of SPA. Sure enough, naloxone also partially, not fully, blocked SPA, while it had no effects of its own. We knew our result was exciting, although we were not sure exactly why. Good instincts, however, are important to research.

At the time, in 1971, Liebeskind was on sabbatical in Paris, working with Denise Albé-Fessard, a great figure in the history of pain research. Her husband, Alfred Fessard, was a member of the French National Academy. I wrote to Liebeskind and told him about my naloxone findings, and he said, "We ought to publish this in a hurry."

Our 1972 paper in *Comptes Rendus*, the proceedings of the French National Academy of Sciences, described our findings that the opiate antagonist naloxone blocked SPA. We concluded with a bold statement that these results suggested "the analgesias produced by electrical stimulation and by the injection of morphine not only act in a common site, the periaqueductal gray, but are caused by the same mechanism" (Akil et al. 1972). We were postulating a mechanism that could be caused by electrical stimulation, but was natural to the brain. Could our electrical currents be releasing something opiate-like in the brain, given that it was blockable by an opiate antagonist?

I presented this work in my first scientific talk, at the International Congress of Pharmacology meeting in San Francisco in 1972. In my 10-minute presentation I described the monoaminergic data, showing the parallels to morphine, and then the naloxone data. At the end of my talk, the first question came from a man with a thick accent, who asked, "Are you saying you can cure pain?" I said, "No," and explained that, of course, one cannot use the word "pain" for animals; one can only report a lack of pain responses or a decrease in nociception. He responded, "Only God can cure pain. You are going to burn in hell!" He then started yelling at me, and security came and pulled him out. While he was being physically dragged backwards from the large auditorium, he kept repeating, "You're burning in hell." That was the first scientific question addressed to me in my professional career. This man had walked into the meeting off the streets of San Francisco, and it was just my luck that he listened to my talk.

The second person to ask me a question was an interesting-looking elderly gentleman who was sitting up front and who also had a strong accent. By then I was really scared. He said, "How do you think this is happening with the naloxone?" I replied: "I really don't know, but I think the effect we are getting is very similar to morphine, whatever it is that we are doing." His face bore a thoughtful look as he sat down. Dozens of questions were then asked. Several prominent opiate researchers drilled me about the details of our experiments. I became even more nervous, because I did not understand the reasons for the significant pressure. Indeed, inquiries continued after the meeting, including an extensive telephone call from another extremely prominent scientist, Avram Goldstein.

I finally got off the dais, and then realized that the person who had asked me the second question was Hans Kosterlitz. I was told afterwards that he was very interested in our work; he was sure the brain had an opiate receptor, and was working to discover the reason for its presence. What was it a receptor for? Surely, it was not simply there to recognize the plant-derived opiates. We had provided him with the first physiological evidence for the existence of an opiate-like factor in the brain that might interact with the opiate receptors. These findings were important because evidence to the contrary had been discouraging. Typically, naloxone given to a quiescent animal produced no observable behavioral effects. These observations contrasted to the dramatic effects of naloxone in reversing the effects of exogenous opiate drugs (heroin, morphine). The absence of a naloxone effect in the normal animal had been taken as evidence of absence of any opiate-like activity in the brain. Our results showed that this system had to be activated first (in this case electrically), and naloxone would then be effective. After hearing my paper, Kosterlitz was concerned that we might be good biochemists who would attempt to purify this opiate-like brain substance and thus "beat him to the punch." As psychologists, however, we had absolutely no idea how to do this.

After I completed my Ph.D. with Liebeskind, I had to wait a year before beginning a postdoctoral position because my husband was finishing his medical degree at Tulane University. I went to Tulane and worked with a neurosurgeon, Don Richardson, who had read some of our work and was interested in determining whether our findings could be applied to patients suffering from intractable pain. For the first time, I was able to see how brain stimulation works in a human being who can talk and describe feelings and sensations resulting from the current. We had come full circle to the original studies of brain stimulation and central pain, except the purpose now was pain relief. The study participants were cancer patients or other pain patients who had become completely tolerant of medication and resistant to standard treatment and who were suffering a great deal.

Richardson wanted to find other ways to intervene, so he started lowering electrodes into the posterior thalamic region, part of the system that we had shown was capable of inhibiting pain. If we went all the way to the periaqueductal gray, it was clear that numerous autonomic side effects made the patients very uncomfortable. So Richardson backed up and found a site near the posterior aspect of the paraventricular nucleus of the thalamus, where the patients tolerated the stimulation very well. For a few days, external electrodes would be connected to a Medtronic stimulation device. I worked with the patients to figure out the right stimulation parameters. If we felt that the stimulation therapy was workable and useful, we implanted the whole system with a silver-dollar-sized receiver unit. Then, if the patient had pain, he or she would put the stimulation device on the chest and try it. Surprisingly, the stimulation was very effective for many patients and gave them pain relief at times when nothing else worked (Richardson and Akil 1977).

During the course of this work, I learned more about opiate analgesia in pain patients. Even though the Tulane patients were on high dosages of opiate drugs, to the point of being completely tolerant, withdrawing the medications was not a traumatic experience for them. They were dependent; when they stopped taking opiates, they felt as if they had influenza for a few days and then they were fine. They did not want or seek opiates and were happy to discontinue the drugs due to all the side effects. The only patients who wanted to continue taking opiates had prior addiction problems and were already drug abusers. It appeared to me that the pain-relieving properties of the opiates and their addictive properties were separable, and that electrical stimulation in the gray areas primarily mimicked their ability to inhibit pain.

During this era of the early 1970s, it became clearer that we needed more detailed information on the opiates. In the late 1960s and early 1970s, opiates were strange territory to the outsider who did not follow the research in the major laboratories. The Symposia on Narcotic and Analgesic Drugs featured many papers on a bewildering number of agonists and antagonists: University of Michigan researchers were doing characterizations, Kosterlitz was looking at the neuromuscular junction and at visceral bioacids, Goldstein was investigating opiate tolerance, and so on.

By 1971, Goldstein and his colleagues had made their first attempts to identify an opiate receptor in the brain. Kosterlitz had confirmed opiate receptors in the gut and in the mouse vas deferens. The Goldstein laboratory had devised a thoughtful scheme for demonstrating these receptors, but encountered serious background problems. Only 2% of what they measured was specific; the rest was background noise. While the study suffered from these technical difficulties, it opened the door to a strategy that others later used successfully.

At that point, several now-famous scientists entered into the picture. One was Solomon Snyder, who was at Johns Hopkins with a laboratory next door to Pedro Cuatrecasas, who had done important basic molecular work on insulin receptors. Snyder wanted to carry that perspective to the opiates. A landmark of the Snyder laboratory is to identify the appropriate pharmacological tools for discovery; thus, they attacked the problem by using an opiate ligand with a higher specific activity for the binding studies. His colleague and graduate student was Candace Pert. In a paper in *Science* that received a great deal of attention, Snyder and Pert (1973) clearly demonstrated the presence of opiate receptors in nervous tissue of the types that we have come to expect for a brain distribution of a neural receptor.

Simultaneously, Eric Simon's laboratory, with Hiller and Edelman, also published a paper in the *Proceedings of the National Academy of Sciences* in which they reported using a different ligand, radiolabeled etorphine, to identify opiate bindings in the brain (Simon et al. 1973). Lars Terenius was in fact the first person to accomplish this feat (Terenius 1973), but he had the bad luck to publish in a more obscure journal. In 1972 he had independently conducted the earliest and most complete work on the presence of opiate receptors in the brain, but it did not become public knowledge until 1973— an amazing year for the recognition of opiate receptors in the brain.

The story now moves to the endorphins. On May 19, 1974, the Neuroscience Research Program (NRP) convened a meeting in Boston co-chaired by Snyder and Steve Mathysse from Harvard University and Massachusetts General Hospital. The select group of invited attendees comprised a *Who's Who* of opiate research at the time. Among them were Bill Martin, the head of the testing site at the U.S. Public Health Service Hospital in Kentucky, as well as Avram Goldstein, Eric Simon, Lars Terenius, Candace Pert, E. Leong Way, John Hughes, Hans Kosterlitz, Floyd Bloom, Leslie Iversen, Arnold Mandel, and a few others. Several attendees—Gavril Pasternak, Ian Creese, and I—were young and unknown. We were the scribes, the ones who took notes during the meeting and helped synthesize them into a book of collected papers; we were required to be intelligent condensers of the drafts presented.

It was the most amazing meeting in my life because we all sat in a relatively small room, facing one other. Everyone was talking about opiate receptor binding, in itself exciting. Toward the end of the meeting, Hughes rose and said: "There are noradrenergic, cholinergic, serotonergic, and GABAergic neurotransmitters. I shall now complicate the picture by suggesting the existence of morphinergic transmission."

He talked about studies, using the guinea pig model that Kosterlitz had developed, showing that brain extract derived from the thousands of grams of midbrain tissue (the SPA-active regions) would inhibit contractions of the guinea pig ileum as if it were morphine. The most important test was that naloxone blocked the effect of the brain extract. If the researchers bathed the ileum with naloxone, they initially reversed a small percentage of the effect of the brain extract. As they continued to purify the brain extract, naloxone reversed an increasingly large percentage until it completely blocked the effect of the extract. This naloxone reversibility was the key pharmacological proof that the extracted material was an opiate-like substance that interacted with the opiate receptor. Hughes and Kosterlitz had not yet named their newly discovered substance and at the NRP meeting simply called the extract substance X, or morphine-like substance. They did not yet know its biochemical composition.

Between that May meeting and December, Hughes and Kosterlitz teamed up with Morgan and Morris and identified the two substances, not as true opiate alkaloid-like substances like the extracts of the poppy, but as pentapeptides—peptides made of five amino acids each, which they named leucine and methionine enkephalin (Hughes et al. 1975). It was amazing that they were peptides—tyr-gly-gly-phe-met or tyr-gly-gly-phe-leu—not simple molecules like morphine.

Between 1975 and 1984, the number of publications on endorphins rose dramatically. Only a small portion dealt with pain. The rest focused on the biology, anatomical location, and function of these peptides. Many meetings were held and many influential scientists moved into the field. It was seen as a new era marked by the emergence of a new class of transmitters that would require a different level of biological understanding.

After my work at Tulane with Richardson, I moved as a postdoctoral fellow to the laboratory of Jack Barchas at Stanford University. My interest had broadened from a focus on analgesia to a desire to understand the function and regulation of the endogenous opioid peptides. What do they do physiologically, assuming that they are not simply released by the highly artificial electrical stimulation we had used? One hypothesis was that endorphins were important for coping with unusual demands on the organism, especially in times of stress. Thus, at Stanford, we characterized a new phenomenon we termed "stress-induced analgesia." We showed that a stressed animal became insensitive to noxious stimuli, and that this response appeared at least in part to be mediated by endorphins because it was preventable by the administration of naloxone (Madden et al. 1977). Subsequent research confirmed both opioid and non-opioid components of stress-induced analgesia. In one of those interesting coincidences in science, both the Liebeskind and Mayer laboratories were concurrently doing parallel studies to characterize the nature and complexities of stress-induced analgesia.

The most interesting questions at that time were: What are the biological synthetic histories of these endorphins? Where are they coming from? Why are there two enkephalins? It was known by then, from work on insulin and other peptide hormones, that the body manufactures peptides by processing larger molecules, i.e., protein precursors. The impetus was great to understand more about the biochemical origins of the opiate-like peptides, which became known as either endogenous opioids or endorphins. In their original enkephalin paper, Hughes and his coworkers had pointed out that the sequence of methionine enkephalin was embedded in the sequence of another peptide, termed β-lipotropin (β-LPH). They wondered whether β-LPH was the precursor to met-enkephalin, and if so, whether a parallel leu-enkephalin precursor existed. Researchers began peptide extraction work and isolated numerous pieces of peptides of varying lengths, all containing the tyr-gly-gly-phe-met or tyr-gly-gly-phe-leu motif of the enkephalins at their amino terminus, with various C-terminal extensions.

Beyond the two enkephalins that were identified by Hughes, Kosterlitz, and their colleagues, a new peptide, termed β-endorphin, attracted great interest. Beta-endorphin was identified by C.H. Li and colleagues at the University of California San Francisco, the same scientific group that had previously identified β-LPH, ACTH, and growth hormone. Li had a powerful peptide and hormone sequencing laboratory that was in competition with the laboratories of Roger Guillemin at the Salk Institute and Andrew Schally at Tulane University. At one point it was estimated that Li's laboratory had characterized something like 80% of the known large peptide hormones.

Li was interested in comparative peptide biology. He liked to study the brains of unusual animals and, several years prior to the discovery of the enkephalins, he had inadvertently identified the sequence of β-endorphin. Li had an Iraqi postdoctoral colleague who sent him camel pituitaries so that he could compare the structure of β-LPH in camels to the known structures of this hormone in other species. In Iraq, camel brains are not well preserved, so instead of extracting full β-lipotropin from the pituitary, he obtained what appeared to be a fragment that started with the sequence tyr-gly-gly-phe-met at its amino terminus and was only 31 amino acids in length (compared to about 90 for β-lipotropin). The substance lay ignored in Li's laboratory until the discovery of the enkephalins. The enkephalin amino acid sequence was embedded into the camel pituitary fragment, so it was reasonable to think that a particular precursor protein would encode for a long sequence that would include β-lipotropin as a peptide precursor or intermediate, and then an enzyme would liberate met-enkephalin. Thus, according to this view, the β-endorphin fragment would only be part of the synthetic pathway of the enkephalins.

Several groups showed, however, that β-endorphin itself had extremely potent biological activity and produced much longer-lasting analgesia than did the enkephalins. Some argued that β-endorphin was the real opioid and that met-enkephalin and leu-enkephalin were merely breakdown products. Hughes suggested that β-endorphin was a pituitary hormone and would therefore be expected to have longer-lasting effects relative to neurotransmitters such as the enkephalins. Regardless of which substance was the "real product," the question remained: Given the above scenario, what about leucine-enkephalin? Did it have a precursor molecule that contained a β-lipotropin or β-endorphin with a leucine in position 5, from which leu-enkephalin could be liberated? Thus, by the late 1970s, many fundamental questions remained about the enkephalins and their relationship to β-endorphin and β-lipotropin. Interestingly, the resolution of these issues came from an unexpected source—neuroanatomy.

Stanley Watson, my husband, and I were now in Barchas' laboratory at Stanford. Floyd Bloom had moved to the Salk Institute and was collaborating with Roger Guillemin, who had become interested in the endorphins. We, at the same time as Bloom's group, developed antibodies and used anatomical clues to determine whether β-endorphin and the enkephalins were biologically connected or were unrelated. We discovered that β-endorphin could indeed be found in the pituitary gland and in the intermediate and anterior lobes, but not in the posterior lobe. We found no enkephalin there. In contrast, we could localize enkephalin in brain regions that lacked β-endorphin. It appeared that the two enkephalins occurred together in the body and that β-endorphin was located in other sites. This discovery, of course, led to a significant revision of the idea that met-enkephalin was derived from β-endorphin, or that leu- and met-enkephalin were necessarily derived from separate precursors.

Our 1978 paper in *Nature* reported the existence of two separate opioid peptide systems and mapped the anatomical distribution of β-endorphin and enkephalins (Watson et al. 1978). The Bloom laboratory performed similar studies at the same time and reached identical conclusions (Bloom et al. 1978). Interestingly, the pathway for β-endorphin almost completely overlapped the sites of stimulation-produced analgesia. We were able to show that the brain area that we had stimulated in human subjects was rich with β-endorphins. Moreover, we demonstrated that the analgesic electrical stimulation releases β-endorphin into the cerebrospinal fluid of human patients. This work nicely brought together the SPA story and the endorphin story, particularly the β-endorphin chapter.

In closing, I would like to briefly review how quickly the field moved into much broader biochemical and neurobiological areas. First, β-lipotropin, a precursor of β-endorphin, turned out to be part of a fascinating molecule that also encodes a stress hormone, adrenocorticotrophic hormone (ACTH), and melanocortin, a peptide that modulates appetite and sexual responsiveness, among other functions. This peptide, termed pro-opiomelanocortin (POMC), was the first mammalian gene to be cloned, and is the prototypical peptide precursor for studying the biosynthesis of peptidergic signaling molecules.

From the slew of peptides isolated over the years emerged another major finding—they could all be assigned to three distinct genes that are now called pro-opiomelanocortin, pro-enkephalin, and prodynorphin. Pro-enkephalin encodes both methionine and leucine enkephalin, the two peptides that Hughes had originally identified. Prodynorphin encodes a large family first identified by Goldstein. All three precursor genes give rise to many peptide products, all sharing that tyr-gly-gly-phe motif, followed by either leu or met, and then, for many, an extended sequence of amino acids. Each of these peptides has a particular distribution and set of actions in the brain. We have learned that the endorphins and the biologically related molecules are released in various combinations, which suggests that transmission at an opioid synapse may involve not a "go-no-go" signal, but rather a complex neurochemical sentence as a means of synaptic communication.

The opioid receptors—κ, δ, and μ—were first pharmacologically identified, followed by characterization of their interactions with the endogenous opioid peptides. That only three existed given the identified range of opioid peptide messengers was surprising. The convergence of many peptides on a small family of receptors remains an intriguing question in the field. While we had learned a great deal about opioids and their receptors, and had an unmatched array of opioid agonists and antagonists with various selectivities for the various receptors, we still lacked the molecular structure of the receptor proteins. Not until December 1992 was the first opioid receptor cloned simultaneously by Christopher Evans at UCLA and Brigitte Kieffer in Strasbourg, France (Evans et al. 1992; Kieffer et al. 1992).

Not until the 1990s did all the components of the system come together so that we could fully explore the molecular biology, anatomy, and function of the endogenous opioids. It was fitting that one of the last critical elements in completing this system, the cloning of an opioid receptor, occurred in the very institution in which Liebeskind and his students had first demonstrated the physiological functioning of brain endorphins. All the key elements of the system were then in hand, and the day of the endorphins had finally dawned.

REFERENCES

Akil H, Mayer DJ. Antagonism of stimulation-produced analgesia by p-CPA, a serotonin synthesis inhibitor. *Brain Res* 1972; 44:692–697.

Akil H, Mayer DJ, Liebeskind JC. Comparison in the rat between analgesia induced by stimulation of periaqueductal gray matter and morphine analgesia. *C R Hebd Seances Acad Sci D Sci Nat* 1972; 274:3603–3605.

Bloom F, Battenberg E, Rossier J, Ling N, Guillemin R. Neurons containing beta-endorphin in rat brain exist separately from those containing enkephalin: immunocytochemical studies. *Proc Natl Acad Sci USA* 1978; 75:1591–1595.

Cheney DL, Goldstein A. The effect of p-chlorophenylalanine on opiate-induced running, analgesia, tolerance and physical dependence in mice. *J Pharmacol Exp Ther* 1971; 177:309–315.

Evans CJ, Keith Jr DE, Morrison H, Magendzo K, Edwards RJ. Cloning of a delta opioid receptor by functional expression. *Science* 1992; 258:1952–1955.

Goldberg J. *Anatomy of a Scientific Discovery*. Toronto: Bantam Books, 1988.

Hughes J, Smith TW, Kosterlitz H, et al. Identification of two related pentapeptides from the brain with potent opiate agonist activity. *Nature* 1975; 278:577–580.

Kieffer BL, Befort K, Gaveriaux-Ruff C, Hirth CG. The delta-opioid receptor: cloning of a cDNA by expression cloning and pharmacological characterization. *Proc Natl Acad Sci USA* 1992; 89:12048–12052.

Madden J, Akil H, Barchas JD. Stress-induced parallel changes in central opioid levels and pain responsiveness in the rat. *Nature* 1977; 266:358–360.

Mayer DJ, Wolfle TL, Akil H, Carder B, Liebeskind JC. Analgesia from electrical stimulation in the brainstem of the rat. *Science* 1971; 174:1351–1354.

Reynolds DV. Surgery in the rat during electrical analgesia induced by focal brain stimulation. *Science* 1969; 164:444.

Richardson DE, Akil H. Pain reduction by electrical brain stimulation in man. Part 1: Acute administration in periaqueductal and periventricular sites. *J Neurosurg* 1977; 47:178–183.

Simon EJ, Hiller JM, Edelman I. Stereospecific binding of the potent narcotic analgesic (3H) etorphine to rat-brain homogenate. *Proc Natl Acad Sci USA* 1973; 70:1947–1949.

Snyder SH, Pert CB. Opiate receptor: demonstration in nervous tissue. *Science* 1973; 179:1011–1014.

Terenius L. Characteristics of the 'receptor' for narcotic analgesics in synaptic plasma membrane fraction from rat brain. *Acta Pharmacol Toxicol* 1973; 33:377–384.

Tsou K, Zhang CS. Studies on the site of analgesic action of morphine by intracerebral micro-injection. *Scientia Sinica* 1964; 13:1099–1109.

Watson SJ, Akil H, Richard CW III, Barchas JD. Evidence for two separate opiate peptide neuronal systems. *Nature* 1978; 275:226–228.

Correspondence to: Huda Akil, PhD, Departments of Neuroscience and Psychiatry and Mental Health Research Institute, 205 Zina Pitcher Place, University of Michigan, Ann Arbor, MI 48109-0720, USA. Email: akil@umich.edu.

Opioids and Pain Relief: A Historical Perspective,
Progress in Pain Research and Management, Vol.
25, edited by Marcia L. Meldrum, IASP Press,
Seattle, © 2003.

8

Taking the Myths out of the Magic: Establishing the Use of Opioids in the Management of Cancer Pain

Christina Faull and Alexander Nicholson

*Department of Palliative Care, University Hospital,
Birmingham, United Kingdom*

Imagine if you will a December day in London in the early 1960s. Let's take a walk down Wimpole Street, a grand but relatively quiet street next to Harley Street. Most portico doorways display shiny brass plaques with the names of nationally and internationally renowned doctors. We arrive at No. 1 and enter the lush, intimidating interior of the Royal Society of Medicine (RSM), established in 1805 as the "Medical and Chirurgical Society of London." The home of the RSM is an awe-inspiring mixture of a club and a temple.

Today the surgical section of the society is meeting to discuss "The Management of Intractable Pain." Members, almost all men, are arriving in their cashmere overcoats, pinstripe suits, shiny black shoes, and hats. Some have even traveled from Ireland on the overnight ferry-train. There is a London pea-souper fog, so many who wanted to come are delayed or have sent their apologies. Cicely Saunders, one of today's speakers, arrives just in time. She has returned in this treacherous weather from a trip to Warsaw, arriving on one of the last planes to land at Heathrow airport.

Joseph Buford Pennybacker, a neurosurgeon from the Radcliffe Infirmary in Oxford, is the first to speak. His opening statement, "I am not certain how far we can get in discussing intractable pain because volumes have been written on the subject and it is still very much with us," would not appear to set a hopeful tone for the event (Pennybacker 1963). The second speaker, John W. Dundee, Professor of Anaesthetics at Queen's University in Belfast, is followed by Saunders.

Tradition has it that, for any physician, addressing a meeting of surgeons is an intimidating experience. Imagine how much more this applies to Saunders who, having completed her house jobs (equivalent to American internship) only 3 years ago, is now working in a place probably unknown to most of these surgeons, St. Joseph's Hospice, in the poor East End of London. She will be talking about death and dying, and therefore about the patients whom surgeons often see as their failures. Furthermore, she is about to contradict several of the myths believed to be true by the vast majority of the audience. She is going to argue that what they have been taught, what they teach, and what they do is wrong. This is a seminal talk for Saunders and for cancer pain control. Although she has recalled how unaware she was of the originality of her work, she was about to start a revolution. As she recounted later, "The fundamentals of therapeutics I believe remain as I wrote in 1963" (Saunders 1996).

The magic of pain relief with opiates had of course been known for centuries. But in this RSM talk, Saunders fired at four myths that at that time were accepted doctrine for the use of opiates. She explained that evidence from her studies of patients indicated that opiates were not addictive for patients with pain from advanced cancer; that regular giving of opiates did not lead to addiction, nor did it cause a major problem of tolerance; that oral morphine was effective; and that it worked not by causing indifference to the pain, but by relieving the pain.

In her talk, Saunders challenged Dundee, the previous speaker, who had said:

> Opinions vary as to whether drugs should be given "as required" or on a fixed time basis. If the latter intervals are slightly shorter than the expected duration of the analgesic, the pain relief will be greater, for it is easier to prevent pain than relieve it when it has occurred. This, however, can lead to the development of tolerance and should be reserved for the terminal stages of malignancy. (Dundee 1963)

He also said, "It is desirable to maintain patients on oral therapy for as long as possible. ... This limits the number of established drugs to levorphanol, methadone and dihydrocodeine." (Dundee 1963). Clearly, in his opinion, oral morphine was not effective.

What was it that Saunders had to say? She spoke about 900 patients with cancer. That in itself was a stunning context. Pennybacker's references were to "some patients," while Dundee related the analysis of 333 cases, of whom 117 had cancer. All of Saunders' 900 patients were thought to have a prognosis of less than 3 months. They were *dying* patients; this was the first ever such series. Few people had systematically observed dying patients prior to Saunders' work. Several eminent late 19th- and early 20th-century authors like William Munk (1887) and Herbert Snow (1896) had recounted anecdotal reports and written with the style "in their experience." Exton-Smith (1961) had reported on the terminal illness of 220 geriatric patients, of whom about 145 had significant pain. Apart from Snow's work, few observations were available about the needs of those dying from cancer.

Saunders spoke at the RSM in her capacity as a member of the pharmacology department at St. Mary's Hospital Medical School, but the work presented was the result of observation rather than scientifically rigorous testing. She used her opening paragraphs to increase the power of her remarks by making it very clear how unsuitable the model of the controlled clinical trial was to her workplace and patient group:

> We have not found that controlled clinical trials are suitable either in this setting or with this particular group of patients ... they have many symptoms, they need a variety of drugs as well as analgesics and their condition is deteriorating, often rapidly. (Saunders 1963)

She also challenged the traditional physical, biomedical approach to managing disease, the approach that would have been familiar and safe to her surgical audience, by introducing a holistic style to the management strategy. "It is not possible to treat pain in isolation for we have to consider the whole person" (Saunders 1963). She made reference to the environment and its impact on the therapeutic outcome: "I am well aware that this is a specialized setting and how much the atmosphere, which is a fundamental part of treatment, is created by the nuns and their nurses" (Saunders 1963). By her very honesty, and by her forthright declaration of the limitations on research conducted in the hospice setting, she preempted skeptics in the audience from belittling the importance of her enormous case series by arguing that such work was not of the quality expected from a prestigious department of pharmacology.

Saunders reported that for 70% of the patients in St. Joseph's Hospice, the main problem was pain; thus she confirmed everyone's worst fears about advanced cancer. Perhaps a gloom came over the audience at this point. No doubt vivid memories of distressed patients came into their minds. What Saunders said next would have startled many: "What I say is so simple that I would be diffident about it if I did not know that it worked and that various students on the many teaching rounds that come to St. Joseph's always remark that our patients are alert and cheerful, as well as free from pain" (Saunders 1963).

This must have been a shocking statement. "Alert" and "cheerful": This picture correlated neither with the general public's nor the doctors' images of the dying patient, nor with their image of the patient on opiates. Such patients, they thought, should be in agony, miserable or comatose, or exhibiting uncontrollable behaviors due to addiction. Saunders went on further to challenge her listeners' preconceptions:

> We are convinced that it is this routine (regular oral giving) that enables us and other such homes to give the same dose of opiates, for weeks and months on end ... Patients may indeed be physically dependent on the drugs but tolerance and addiction are not problems to us, even with those who stay the longest. ... Our patients do not talk of their indifference to pain but of the absence of pain. (Saunders 1963)

Textbooks from the era give us some insight in to how controversial Saunders' 1962 talk was. Laurence and Moulton (1960) discussed the two mechanisms of analgesia: first, a reduction in the patient's ability to perceive the sensation of pain, and second, an alteration of the appreciation of the sensation so that it was no longer unpleasant. They went on to note that: "Unfortunately all the most potent drugs act in both ways so that although pain may be relieved, the patient cannot be considered to be mentally entirely normal whilst under their influence." Other standard texts observed: "Some physicians believe that he [the patient] should learn to endure pain, with the hope that it may lessen rather than be put on narcotics with the impression that it is hopeless and he might just as well be an addict" (Dock 1950). "Intractable pain due to incurable disease such as metastatic carcinoma is one of the most difficult of therapeutic problems. As a rule, one resorts to narcotic drugs because of their strong analgesic action, and habituation is accepted as the lesser of two evils" (Harrison et al. 1966).

In the foreword to the American text *The Management of Pain in Cancer*, Cole (1956) writes: "Unfortunately, practically all the drugs that are really effective in controlling pain are habit producing and therefore must be used sparingly." Cole himself indicated that opiates should be used relatively freely in patients in the last few days of life. The insistence of other contributors that opiates should be severely rationed in all other circumstances illustrates how radical Saunders' thesis was: "Addiction and particularly tolerance are important in the patient with long-term chronic pain. In such instances every effort should be made to put off the use of the potent addicting drug until all other measures have been exhausted" (Schiffrin 1956). Other drugs, which we now know to be addictive, were more freely advocated: "The fear of pain and the individual reaction to pain can also be modified by the use of agents other than analgesics, such as barbiturates, amphetamine and other drugs that affect the emotional plane and sensorium" (Schiffrin 1956). Analgesics were subdivided into nonaddicting drugs and addicting drugs. On addicting drugs, the recommendations in this text were stunningly in opposition to Saunders' methods:

> Tolerance to addicting drugs begins early; in fact, there is good evidence that it is operative after the very first dose. ... The appearance of clinically significant tolerance can be delayed by using the minimal effective dose as infrequently as possible. ... The writing of an order as "1/4 gr morphine q.4 h" is to be deplored. (Schiffrin 1956)

The author also said of morphine: "Given orally, it produces little analgesia, and therefore the parenteral routes are preferred" (Schiffrin 1956).

Widely used general medical text books of the time in the United Kingdom tended to ignore the issues of pain in cancer and the use of opiates. *The Principles and Practice of Medicine: A Textbook for Student Doctors,* first published in 1952 as a summary of Stanley Davidson's lecture notes for Scottish medical students, has one brief entry in the section on disease of the digestive system. "As in the management of other carcinomatous patients, analgesics should be given in sufficient amounts to control pain" (Davidson 1962).

Saunders recalled in 1999 how pain was managed in her early days in hospital as a nurse and social worker:

> I saw patients in pain, I listened to families talking about pain after the patient had gone home. Although we were giving the Brompton cocktail ... it was very much p.r.n. or 4 hourly p.r.n. ... you had to earn your morphine by having pain first. (Saunders 1999)

She has also recalled her introduction of regular giving of morphine when she first went to St. Joseph's Hospice from St. Luke's Home for the Dying Poor in Bayswater, London, a hospice founded by Howard Barrett in 1893, where she had worked as a volunteer nurse. "I was given four patients to look after. I put them on the regular schedule and I got them to keep a diary and it was like waving a wand" (Saunders 1991). "Sister Mary Antonia who was my first warden ... wrote to me a few years ago saying 'I well remember the change from pain full to pain free' by simply taking what they were giving and putting it 4 hourly'" (Saunders 1999). It was her memory of these amazing changes in patients and the impact on nurses and students that made Saunders less diffident as she explained her innovations to the potentially skeptical and hostile surgical audience at the RSM.

What brought Saunders to be able to challenge and change the world of cancer pain management at this time and place? At the age of 44 she was relatively mature and had worked both as a nurse and a social worker. It was through her work with the renowned St. Thomas' Hospital surgeon, Norman

'Pasty' Barrett, that she was persuaded to study medicine. She has recalled his advice to her in the late 1940s: "It is the doctors that desert the dying; there is so much more to be learnt about pain. You'll only be frustrated if you don't do it [improve the care of dying patients] properly and they [doctors] won't listen to you [unless you are a doctor]" (Saunders 1999). A letter to her principal at St. Anne's College in Cambridge explained her motivation:

> I have become more and more aware of the problems of the dying, particularly of the hopeless advanced cases of cancer, and I do think their feeling that they are deserted by the doctors is to some extent justified. I want very badly to try and find out more about the possibilities of alleviating their physical and mental distress and realize I can only do this by becoming a doctor. (Du Boulay 1994)

At the time of the 1962 talk, the library at the RSM had become Saunders' second home. She spent hours there reading about cancer pain management, composing her thoughts, and writing and developing her plans for a new focus on the care of patients with advanced cancer. Saunders recalled that she wrote to an enormous number of people involved in pain management, seeking information and outlining her work at St. Joseph's Hospice. She believed it was probably through her correspondence with Dundee that she was invited to speak at the 1962 meeting. She recalled being excited, but surprisingly not unduly nervous about giving the talk. "I had done a lot of solo singing in my time and that stood me in good stead" (Saunders 2002).

Clark (1998) has discussed many of the factors that influenced Saunders in developing her dream of a model hospice and promoting her vision of a way to improve care for patients with terminal cancer, a vision that was beginning to come to life in 1962. The Certificate of Incorporation for St. Christopher's Hospice, the start needed to bring the dream to fruition, was registered in 1961. This institution would achieve excellence in care, teaching, and research. Her experiences as a volunteer nurse at St. Luke's (1948–1955) and then at St. Joseph's (1958–1965) were important in shaping her thoughts. As a woman with a private income, she was perhaps free to take her vision forward relatively independently of the hierarchy of medicine and the usual subjugation to a need for professional references. No doubt Saunders' strong Christian beliefs, which underpinned her vision, contributed the necessary missionary zeal. Perhaps above all, Saunders was driven by love and by the grief of love lost. Many biographies and oral histories have documented Saunders' relationships with two dying men. As a nurse in 1947, she met David Tasma, who made the famous statement, "I'll be a window in your home." While working at St. Joseph's in 1960, less than 18 months before her RSM talk, she had an intense love affair with Antoni Michniewicz.

Soon after the 1962 presentation at the RSM, Saunders began to develop a new style of lecturing, using individual patient stories to help people "see" by proxy. Pictures of patients accompanied these patient narratives. Even her writing began to take on this new format (Clark 1998). It was not only revolutionary but also highly effective.

Saunders has recalled the regular lectures she presented during 1965–1986 at the London Medical Group, an extracurricular program of lectures for students from London's 12 medical schools, as follows:

> I used to get a packed house every time. It was always what the students wanted. … Talking about stories, but showing a graph that we didn't get escalation and perhaps a histogram of the sort of doses that we were using; and comparing chronic pain with acute, teaching hospital pain. But mainly talking stories on the physical side, the family side, the psychological side and by having done all that you could even tackle the spiritual side without minds closing all round the room. It was giving a voice to the voiceless. … Getting the patient to tell the story, because you can put in some statistics but when you tell the stories that's what moves people. It was really getting the students to think about the whole person. (Saunders 1999)

Saunders often met people who recalled her talks "because on the whole people weren't talking like that. Lots of people talk with slides with people and pictures and so on I think now. It was a bit new when I started." (Saunders 1999)

Saunders had brought from St. Luke's to St. Joseph's the regular giving of oral morphine, but at the time of the RSM talk, she was refining her thoughts about the opiate of choice.

> I would like to add a note on the use of diamorphine. It was given to 42 of our first 500 patients, to women who were nauseated by other opiates and to a few patients who had intolerable feelings of suffocation. It was used so effectively that since then we ceased using almost all other powerful analgesics in its favour. No other drug makes the patient look and feel so comfortable. (Saunders 1962)

The superiority of diamorphine, or heroin, as an analgesic was another myth waiting to be challenged. Its putative clinical prowess perhaps stemmed from its initial launch by Bayer in 1899. "Heroin possesses many advantages over morphine …: 1) it prolongs respiration …; 2) it is not a hypnotic; 3) absence of danger of acquiring the habit," wrote a commentator in the *Boston Medical and Surgical Journal* (Daly 1900). In the mid-1950s, there had been great international debate about the continued medicinal use of diamorphine. The World Health Organization (WHO) issued a bulletin on narcotics in 1953, recommending that all countries ban importation and use of the drug. A 1955 editorial in the *Lancet* suggested that a controlled trial was needed to provide evidence to support or refute a ban of diamorphine (Anonymous 1955), and the U.K. government decided not to follow the WHO recommendations regarding a ban. Only one other country (Belgium) still allowed the medicinal use of diamorphine by 1962.

By the time of Saunders' RSM talk, there was considerable emphasis in the U.K. medical literature on the benefits of diamorphine over morphine. "Heroin is a powerful euphoriant, analgesic, cough and respiratory depressant, and perhaps causes less vomiting than morphine, and greater euphoria with less sleepiness" (Laurence and Moulton 1960). Not all authorities rendered such a positive verdict, however. The *British National Formulary* (BNF) was another influence on the prescribing practices of U.K. doctors. Originally a war formulary, the BNF proved so useful that the Joint Formulary Committee of the British Medical Association and the Royal Pharmaceutical Society continued its production. New editions were produced every 3 years until 1981, when government review mandated a new comprehensive publication, updated every 6 months and distributed free to physicians. When Saunders was researching at St. Joseph's in the early 1960s, the analgesic and antipyretic section of the BNF stated: "Diamorphine is more toxic than morphine and should be used with caution, if at all. It gives rise to less vomiting and constipation than does morphine but has a much greater liability to cause addiction" (British Medical Association 1960).

In a later edition the BNF perpetuated the notion that there were crucial differences between diamorphine and morphine, but in language that would surely have made any doctor or nurse afraid to use the former:

> Analgesia is accompanied by notable mental detachment and by euphoria instead of sedation. ... action by all routes lasts about half as long as morphine. There is much less nausea than with morphine. ... Tolerance develops and diamorphine is the most addictive drug of the series. It should not be used for more than a week or so except in patients where addiction does not matter. The medical use of diamorphine is illegal in some countries, but not in the United Kingdom. (British Medical Association 1963)

Saunders was, as always, keen to test the reality of her enthusiasms. She was perhaps aware that her advocacy of the use of diamorphine rather than morphine would curtail the global potential of her pain control message. Certainly this became clear to her when her beliefs in diamorphine were refuted. When the myth was dispelled, she stated: "What I realized more firmly later was that, if we'd had a magic drug which nobody else could use we'd have had no effect on anybody. Whereas what we could say was that it's not the drug that you use, it's the way that you use it" (Saunders 1999).

When St. Christopher's Hospice opened in 1967, she obtained grants from the Department of Health and Social Security and the Sir Halley Stewart Trust to compare the effects of morphine and diamorphine. Robert Twycross took up the Research Fellowship at St. Christopher's Hospice in 1971 and began work on the comparison studies.

> Saunders believed that diamorphine was better because it was less sedative, caused less nausea and vomiting, and I don't know what else, but she wanted to prove this. Well, as you may know I disproved it, and so in 1976 or maybe sooner at St. Christopher's, we all changed over to [oral] morphine. (Twycross 1999)

During his 5 years at St. Christopher's from 1971 to 1976, Twycross (1976) undertook four key studies that formed the basis for his DM thesis. First he reviewed the experiences of 418 of 500 patients admitted consecutively to St. Christopher's who were prescribed oral diamorphine. This research affirmed Saunders' observations that psychological dependence and tolerance were not practical issues in properly managed patients, and that diamorphine use did not necessarily lead to impairment of mental faculties. Second, he studied a subgroup of 115 patients who had received prolonged diamorphine treatment (between 12 and 44 weeks) and found that tolerance was not inevitable; patients were able to adjust to lower doses as pain levels decreased. Dose reductions were not infrequent, and the median final dose in the subgroup was less than the median maximum dose. Twycross' third project was a randomized double-blind trial comparing oral morphine with oral diamorphine in 196 patients (Twycross 1976).

This study was followed by a randomized, double-blind crossover trial comparing oral morphine with oral diamorphine, entering 699 patients, of whom 146 completed the crossover. It was the first trial of its kind in palliative care in the United Kingdom and broke new ground in presenting a research model with patients who were dying. It remains the largest single-center crossover study of opioid use in patients with cancer-related pain, and when it appeared in *Pain* it was the first such study to be published in a major, widely disseminated journal. These trials demonstrated that oral morphine and oral diamorphine were equally effective analgesics, if the dosage was correctly titrated (Twycross 1977).

In all, Twycross had collated information on 1,313 patients, and Saunders had undertaken 1,100 patient studies. This huge evidence base led both doctors to two irrefutable conclusions. First, the regular giving of an opiate "by the clock" provided good pain relief that did not invariably require steady dose increases over time—that is, patients did not develop tolerance to the drug—and that also did not lead to addiction (psychological dependence). Second, the method of giving—*how* an opiate was used—was more important than *which* opiate was used. This work was to provide a significant evidence base for the cardinal principles of the method of cancer pain relief—the WHO analgesic ladder—endorsed by the WHO in its highly influential publication *Cancer Pain Relief* (1986). The WHO Cancer Pain Relief Program aimed to improve pain management for the estimated 3.5 million people suffering from cancer pain worldwide. The program included government-driven cancer pain relief programs in every country, improved access to controlled drugs, an evidence-based method of cancer pain relief, and education of health care professionals in the assessment and management of cancer pain. The first meeting of an international clinician group to develop the evidence-based method that became the WHO analgesic ladder took place in Milan, Italy, in 1982 (see Swerdlow, this volume).

The work of Saunders and Twycross was highly influential on cancer pain control methods and the teaching of hospice and specialist palliative care teams in the United Kingdom. There was, however, considerable international debate. The studies of Raymond Houde and his team at Sloan-Kettering in New York had found that the relative potency of oral morphine was low and that the development of tolerance was inevitable. In 1979 Houde concluded, therefore, that the oral morphine would have to be escalated to very large, perhaps unfeasibly heavy, doses, and that other drugs were superior or more reliable for oral use. Twycross, on the basis of his studies, argued that the patient's pain could be comfortably controlled on oral morphine without escalation, as long as it was regularly given by the clock. He has recalled:

> The debate, well I think it was ongoing, but you see Ray Houde and company, they were teaching that it was no good, and at the first World Congress on Pain in Florence [1975]. … I couldn't stand it any more, so I strode up to the front when I had the opportunity and drew a few things on the overhead and said what we did, to loud cheers from the Brits in the audience. (Twycross 1999)

The debate, which was at times acrimonious, about the value of oral morphine and to some extent the issue of tolerance continued for over 10 years and influenced the discussions surrounding the development of WHO's cancer pain relief program. Meldrum (Chapter 14) and M.L. Meldrum and D. Clark (unpublished manuscript) have discussed how oral morphine became the suggested drug of choice in the draft WHO manual on cancer pain management. Successful field testing of the draft guidelines gave strong support to this approach.

The WHO field tests were quickly followed by effective trials of the first sustained-release oral morphine compounds (Hanks and Truman 1984). Controlled-release morphine in tablet form had been introduced to the United Kingdom in 1981 by Napp Laboratories as MST Continus. Geoffrey Hanks and his team examined the role of MST Continus in 18 patients with advanced cancer pain, studying those whose pain control had been stable on a regime of 4-hourly morphine sulfate aqueous solution for the previous 7 days (Hanks et al. 1987). (Geoffrey Hanks left the pharmaceutical industry in 1979 to return to clinical medicine and conducted research with Twycross at Sir Michael Sobell House in Oxford during 1979–1983. He subsequently held consultant and teaching posts in palliative care in London before his appointment as Professor of Palliative Medicine at Bristol University in 1993.) This study was one of only three valuable randomized double-blind trials identified in a review of the European experience of controlled-release morphine some 10 years later—a grand total of 49 patients having completed these three trials (Hanks 1989). Hanks' work established that controlled-release and immediate-release oral morphine have equal potency, milligram for milligram, provide effective control of pain, and produce a similar pattern of side effects.

In 1991, Hanks and colleagues surveyed current analgesic practice among U.K. clinicians in a variety of settings—specialist oncology units, teaching hospitals, district general hospitals, and general practice (White et al 1991). Using questionnaires, the team explored doctors' attitudes and knowledge about prescribing strong analgesics. The overall response rate was 42%, presumably representing the more motivated clinicians. Eighty percent or more of respondents were using morphine as the strong opioid analgesic of choice, given by mouth, regularly, in line with WHO recommendations. Controlled-release morphine was more popular among the more recently qualified, but there was considerable confusion about its appropriate use. The most significant findings from this study related to the myths surrounding the use of strong opioids. Concerns about addiction and tolerance were no longer seen as major barriers to the use of these drugs, nor was length of prognosis considered to be a major determining factor in the use of opioid analgesia.

It is interesting and important to focus some attention on the world of laboratory-based opioid research in the United Kingdom around the time these developments were occurring in the clinical field. Since the 1920s efforts had been directed toward the discovery of an analgesic that would be powerfully effective yet nonaddictive, supported by funding from national and private organizations in the United States. The key players in this narrative were provided with the opportunity, and the capital for their research, in part by American funding linked with Richard Nixon's war on drug abuse.

This story concerns highly motivated, very busy individuals forging ahead with work that was almost parallel in its intention to that of the clinicians. During the time that Twycross was a research fellow at St. Christopher's, both the opiate receptor and the endogenous opioids were discovered. The magic of opioid analgesia was thus twice demystified.

> There was a mechanism for explaining how morphine worked. Having a rational basis for something you were doing is far better than just empirically giving a drug that you don't know what it does or how it works. ... The other aspect, far more important than most people think, is that we can explain to people how complex the system is, and that people who have bizarre pain or strange side effects who feel that they may be abnormal, or crazy, can be reassured. (Dickenson 1999)

Hans Kosterlitz and John Hughes were the key players in the discovery of enkephalin. Kosterlitz had studied medicine in Germany where, in the 1930s, tremendous determination was needed to achieve progress in a medical career.

> One was lucky to be allowed to work on the wards and laboratories of a university department. ... I did not receive any remuneration for two or three years. When I obtained my first paid appointment (as an assistant diagnostic radiologist) the clinical and laboratory work in which I was interested had to be done in my spare time. (Kosterlitz 1979)

Following his emigration to the United Kingdom in 1934, he worked as a physiologist at the University of Aberdeen. In 1962, at the time Saunders delivered her RSM talk, Kosterlitz changed direction in his research. Prompted by his observations of the effect of morphine on the autonomic nervous system, he traveled to the United States to become familiar with the field of narcotic analgesia. He visited the laboratories of Julius Axelrod and met Nathan Eddy. These links were formalized in the development of the International Narcotics Research Club in 1969.

In 1968, the University of Aberdeen, recognizing the growing importance of the subject in the medical undergraduate curriculum, had asked Kosterlitz to set up the new department of pharmacology. He was then 65, an age when he would normally have been expected to retire. His acceptance of the commission is another example of the dedication he had shown as a medical student and junior doctor. When he finally retired from the university in 1973, he obtained funding for the directorship of the new Unit for Research on Addictive Drugs (Kosterlitz 1979). Part of the funding for Kosterlitz's new unit came from the U.S. National Institute of Drug Abuse (NIDA). President Nixon introduced several new policy initiatives, including increased research support, in launching his "War on Drugs" in 1971. American concerns had been intensified by the apparent prevalence of narcotic addiction among Vietnam veterans.

John Hughes, a member of Kosterlitz's Department of Pharmacology since 1969, joined him in the new unit. Hughes was not immediately interested in the effect of morphine on physiological systems, but his interest was piqued by the work of a doctoral student. Why should there be morphine receptors in the gut of the guinea pig, the eyelid membrane of the cat, and the vas deferens of the mouse?

In 1972, Huda Akil, a graduate student in John Liebeskind's laboratory at the University of California Los Angeles, presented her work at the International Pharmacology Congress in San Francisco. She showed that electrical stimulation of the periaqueductal area of the rat brain induced profound analgesia, an effect reversible with naloxone (Akil, this volume; Akil et al. 1972). A few delegates at the meeting, including Kosterlitz, concluded that this observation indicated the presence of an endogenous opioid-like substance in the mammalian body. When Hughes subsequently heard about this proposal, it affirmed his new research direction.

Hughes worked initially on extract of rat brain—and a large amount of brain tissue was needed to produce a very little extract. By a fluke he discovered, in January, 1974, that some extracts, stored in the refrigerator, not the freezer, showed convincing evidence of the presence of the substance he was looking for. This exciting moment forced consideration of the practical matter of how to obtain sufficient brain material for further research. Hughes cultivated, with the aid of a bottle or two of whisky, the assistance of a local abattoir with fairly relaxed practices—the place was closed down a year or two later—which allowed the researcher as many pig heads, helpfully cracked open so that he could dissect out the brain tissue, as he desired. His dedication to his quest is evident: up at 5 a.m., cycling through the deserted streets of Aberdeen down to the docks to get dry ice, and back to the abattoir for a 3-hour session on the benches slicing off the cortex of the shelled-out pig brains and freezing the rest on the dry ice. The dry ice container was perched on a conveniently acquired supermarket basket that fitted on the back of the bicycle, keeping the extracts safe on their journey to the drug addiction research laboratories. Here Hughes would spend the rest of the morning grinding the brain tissue into fine powder and extracting the material for analysis (Kosterlitz 1979).

Later that year (1974), 100 members of the International Narcotics Research Club met in Cocoyoc, Mexico. Kosterlitz could not contain his excitement and announced at this meeting his senior researcher's discovery of an endogenous opioid-like substance. He returned triumphantly to Aberdeen to say that Hughes had been invited to attend an upcoming Neuroscience Research Program seminar in Boston that would discuss the opioid receptors and endogenous ligands. Hughes was "incandescent with fury"—indeed it was one of the few times the two ever had fallen out (Tansey and Christie 1997). His anxiety reflected his knowledge of the competitiveness of American scientific research and the risk to their own department of being drawn into an uneven race with substantially better funded transatlantic rivals.

Hughes published his findings in *Brain Research* the following year (1975). He had found a naturally occurring opiate-like substance, but its chemical composition remained to be determined. This piece and the subsequent publication in *Nature* (Hughes et al. 1975) caused enormous scientific and lay interest—such excitement that there was even an article in the *London Times* (1975). The expectations for this scientific breakthrough were tremendous: "Perhaps the most important practical question is whether enkephalin offers the long sought approach to the development of a non-addictive analgesic" (Iverson 1975).

Hughes and Kosterlitz were awarded the Lasker prize in 1978, a prestigious American basic medical research award. The term "endorphin" has since entered common parlance. Hughes' thoughts about the impact of his work are interesting:

> Rather than a black box, you've now got something that you can put in a scientific context, because it was a black box, an absolute black box. So now at least we have a sense that we know that we are doing, probably don't know, but we have a sense, and I think that's important: put it in scientific context. I think for the physician it probably helps. But morphine has such bad press that anything will help. … It always amazes me when I see these terms 'I must stimulate my endorphins' … there aren't many scientific words that reach the popular literature. I think this happened because of holistic medicine. Stimulating your own internal reserves and so on fitted in with all those theories and so fitted with the culture of that time. (Hughes 1999)

Three interesting contrasts become apparent at this point in the story. First we observe that research leading to discovery of the endogenous opioid systems was well funded because of the need to understand the addiction problems that had been a concern since the 1920s and had been particularly highlighted by cases of Vietnam veterans. On the other hand, efforts to refute concerns over addiction in patients with pain were not recognized with this sort of grand initiative or financial support. Saunders, greatest of all advocates for the nonaddicting nature of opioids when used to provide analgesia in the profoundly ill patient, had formulated her experience working at St. Joseph's Hospice, a meagerly funded charitable facility. Her own research efforts were conducted with a marked degree of self-sacrifice and dedication.

The second contrast is a difference between the public style of some key players, reflecting the parts they played in the unfolding drama. A reticent Hughes was closely and carefully questioned at the Boston meeting; efforts made to encourage him to reveal specific scientific details were almost as determined as his own pig brain material extractions. Twycross, a year later, at the first meeting of the International Association for the Study of Pain in Florence, could not have been more different. He strode to the front of the auditorium at the first opportunity and drew an outline representation of British practice at the time, to emphasize and advertise the convictions born of clinical experience. His evangelism was rewarded with cheers from British colleagues in the audience. Hughes was reserved, cautious, minimalist, seeking to preserve a little of the lead in the race and so to make further discoveries ahead of the pack, typical of the scientist eager to pursue a discovery further. Twycross, by contrast, was driven to inform the world, to urge change in clinical practice, and to improve the experience of pain for the greatest number of patients.

The third contrast concerns the speed with which the new discoveries changed behavior and activity. Endogenous opioid system discoveries generated excitement and extremely rapid changes in thinking. Stephen Locke (editor of the *British Medical Journal* from 1975 to 1991), speaking at the Wellcome Witness Seminar in 1996, had a theory that new knowledge takes 36 months to get into publication from conceptualization. Dissemination through the "invisible college," however—the author's peers, the paper's referees, and the "old boy network"—starts to influence ideas after as little as 18 months, perhaps even sooner (Tansey and Christie 1997). Jack Morley, of the Pain Relief Foundation at Walton Hospital in Liverpool, has recalled:

> Kosterlitz and John Hughes up in Aberdeen rang me up about the search for an endogenous opiate. We had quite a good pharmacology group in my department ... immediately set up opioid assays. ... We must have made about 5–600 enkephalin analogues within weeks. Hans and John were most interested of course and we kept them informed about what was going on. (Morley 1999)

As the 1970s gave way to the 1980s, the discovery of enkephalin and endogenous opioid receptors had become established in pharmacology teaching and the scientific literature, but for the clinicians, and especially in clinical textbooks, accepted wisdom evolved more slowly. Patrick Wall, when asked to reflect on whether these discoveries had influenced cancer pain management, stated: "Astonishingly not." And to prove the point further, he waved his hand at a new textbook, hot off the press (Stein 1999), and observed: "In this book here the basic people are full of subdivisions of receptors and compounds that affect things. You read the clinical chapters and there's not a mention of any of this" (Wall 1999). Perhaps even more surprisingly, there was remarkably little impact of the scientific events on the clinicians at the time. Twycross recalled in 1999: "What impact did it have on me? Well, scientifically it was interesting but I'm not sure that it had any real impact ... any practical importance." Saunders, always much more the social and spiritual scientist, said: "I didn't really pick up on that" (Saunders 1999). This obliviousness seems to have been matched by the absence of any direct attention to the clinicians' work by the scientists. Saunders met Kosterlitz through her work on the Medical Research Council (MRC):

> I remember having Kosterlitz here (at St. Christopher's) ... I was on the MRC as a 'lay' member for 4 years ... I remember us talking in our study centre and I'm sure it was Kosterlitz who was saying that he just didn't know that clinically you could use the opioids without the tolerance that he could produce in the lab with his animals. (Wall 1999)

MRC annual reports indicate that this meeting would have taken place sometime between 1977 and 1980. Despite the passage of 18 years since Saunders spoke of clinical findings at the RSM, the addiction and tolerance myths relating to clinical practice still prevailed in the scientific community. Wall stated in 1999 that he still observed evidence of the scientist/clinician divide:

> The basic pharmacologists are still fascinated with habituation and the need for a rising dose, and they're still working on up-regulation of the receptors and so on. It's astonishing to look at the basic pharmacologists still working on what isn't a problem. It is all tied up in something of a hysterical approach. All to do with as soon as you mention narcotics, thinking of social addicts and imagining all the problems of narcotics which is not something that you see in a Hospice for example. (Wall 1999)

Despite these contrasts underlying the provision and scale of resources for the work, the launch style of certain researchers, and the rate of exchange of ideas within and between the scientific and clinical communities, the determination and application of the players in this drama could not have been more alike.

The process by which the myths of opioid use in cancer pain management have been dispelled is fascinating. Kosterlitz's visit to St. Christopher's changed his perceptions of pain, opiates, and addiction. The field testing of oral morphine in line with the draft version of *Cancer Pain Relief* guidelines did more to change practice than Twycross was able to achieve through presentation and debate at meetings. Use of patient narratives influenced the practice and attitudes of individual clinicians much more than did statistics and traditional textbook discussion of evidence or opinion. Only seeing is believing, and only believing changed behavior.

What has "seeing" the endogenous opioid system contributed to this process? New understanding of pain and new models of analgesia, but essentially no change in the clinical armamentarium. Perhaps seeing that drugs such as morphine and diamorphine mimic a natural system, seeing that there is a biomedical model for their mode of action, has allayed some of the fears about their use and helped change clinical practice.

Thirty years after the first major teaching exposition, Hanks and colleagues revealed that the majority of doctors responding to a U.K. survey chose to use regular morphine or diamorphine given orally, titrating the dose against pain severity with no arbitrary upper limit for severe pain in patients with cancer (White et al. 1991). Fears of respiratory depression and addiction and a relatively long prognosis no longer appeared to be deterrents to the use of strong analgesics in these patients.

The magic is stronger than ever, even though the trick is now understood—but where are the myths?

ACKNOWLEDGMENTS

This research was supported by a Wellcome Trust Research Fellowship.

REFERENCES

Akil H, Mayer DJ, Liebeskind JC. Comparison in the rat between analgesia induced by stimulation of periaqueductal gray matter and morphine analgesia. *CR Hebdomadaires Seances Acad Sci D Sci Nat* 1972; 274:3603–3605.

Anonymous. Heroin. Editorial. *Lancet* 1955; I:1311.

British Medical Association. *British National Formulary,* 4th ed. London: British Medical Association, 1960, p 18.

British Medical Association. *British National Formulary,* 5th ed. London: British Medical Association, 1963, p 25.

Clark D. Originating a movement: Cicely Saunders and the development of St. Christopher's Hospice, 1957–1967. *Mortality* 1998; 3:43–63.

Cole W. Foreword. In: Schiffrin MJ (Ed). *The Management of Pain in Cancer*. Chicago: Year Book, 1956.

Daly JRL. A clinical study of heroin. *Boston Med Surg J* 1900; 142(February22):190–192.

Davidson LSP (Ed). *The Principles and Practice of Medicine: Notes for Scottish Medical Students,* 6th ed. Edinburgh: Churchill Livingstone, 1962.

Dickenson A. Oral History Interview, conducted by Faull C, January 1999.

Dock W. Principles of neoplasia. In: Harrison TR, Resnick WR, Wintrobe MM, et al. (Eds). *Principles of Internal Medicine,* 5th ed. New York: McGraw-Hill, 1950, p 290.

Du Boulay S. *Cicely Saunders: The Founder of the Modern Hospice Movement,* 2nd ed. London: Hodder & Stoughton, 1994.

Dundee JW. Remarks. *Proc R Soc Med Section Surgery* 1963; 56:194.

Exton-Smith AN. Terminal illness in the aged. *Lancet* 1961; II:305–308.

Hanks GW. Controlled release morphine (MST Contin) in advanced cancer: the European experience. *Cancer* 1989; 63:2378–2382.

Hanks GW, Truman T. Controlled-release morphine sulphate tablets are effective in twice-daily dosage in chronic cancer pain. In: Wilkes E, Levy J (Eds). *Advances in Morphine Therapy*. London: Royal Society of Medicine, 1984, pp 103–105.

Hanks GW, Twycross RG, Bliss JM. Controlled release morphine tablets; a double-blind trial in patients with advanced cancer. *Anaesthesia* 1987; 42:840–844.

Harrison TR, Adams RD, Bennett IL (Eds). *Principles of Internal Medicine,* 5th ed. New York: McGraw-Hill, 1966.

Houde RW. Systemic analgesics and related drugs: narcotic analgesics. In: Bonica JJ, Ventafridda V (Eds). *International Symposium on Pain of Advanced Cancer,* Advances in Pain Research and Therapy, Vol. 2. New York: Raven Press, 1979, pp 263–273.

Hughes J. Isolation of an endogenous compound from the brain with pharmacological properties similar to morphine. *Brain Res* 1975: 88:295–308.

Hughes J. Oral History Interview, conducted by Faull C, March 1999.

Hughes J, Smith TW, Kosterlitz HW, et al. Identification of two related pentapeptides from the brain with potent agonist activity. *Nature* 1975; 258:577–579.

Iverson L. News and views. *Nature* 1975; 258:567–568.

Kosterlitz HW. The best laid schemes o' mice an' men gang aft agley. *Annu Rev Pharmacol Toxicol* 1979; 19:1–2.

Laurence DR, Moulton R. *Clinical Pharmacology*. London: Churchill, 1960.

London Times. Pharmacology: brain drug like morphine. *London Times* 1975; December:15.

Morley J. Oral History Interview, conducted by Faull C, February 1999.

Munk W. *Euthanasia; or Medical Treatment in and of an Easy Death.* London: Longmans Green & Co., 1887.

Pennybacker J. Opening statement. *Proc R Soc Med Section Surgery* 1963; 56:191.

Royal Society of Medicine. Management of intractable pain. *Proc R Soc Med Section Surgery* 1963; 56:191–197.

Saunders C. Remarks. *Proc R Soc Med Section Surgery* 1963; 56:195–196.

Saunders C. Oral History Interview, conducted by Blythe M, 1991. Wellcome Medical Sciences Video Archive, Library of the Royal College of Physicians.

Saunders C. A personal therapeutic journey. *BMJ* 1996; 313:1600.

Saunders C. Oral History Interview, conducted by Faull C, February 1999.

Saunders C. Oral History Interview, conducted by Faull C, May 2002.

Schiffrin MJ (Ed). *The Management of Pain in Cancer*. Chicago: Year Book, 1956.

Snow H. Opium and cocaine in the treatment of cancerous disease. *BMJ* 1896; II:718–719.

Stein C (Ed). *Opioids in Pain Control: Basic and Clinical Aspects*. Cambridge: Cambridge University Press, 1999.

Tansey EM, Christie DA (Eds). Endogenous opiates. In: *Wellcome Witness to Twentieth Century Medicine,* Vol. I. London: Wellcome Trust, 1997.

Twycross RG. *Studies on the Use of Diamorphine in Advanced Malignant Disease.* DM thesis, Oxford University, 1976.

Twycross RG. Choice of strong analgesic in terminal care: diamorphine or morphine? *Pain* 1977; 3:93–104.

Twycross RG. Oral History Interview, conducted by Faull C, March 1999.

Wall PD. Oral History Interview, conducted by Faull C, January 1999.

White ID, Hoskin PJ, Hanks GW, Bliss JM. Analgesics in cancer pain: current practice and beliefs. *Br J Cancer* 1991; 63:271–274.

World Health Organization. *Cancer Pain Relief.* Geneva: World Health Organization, 1986.

Correspondence to: Alexander Nicholson, MBBS, Specialist Registrar in Palliative Medicine, Compton Hospice, Compton Road West, Wolverhampton WV3 9DH, United Kingdom. Fax: 44-1902-745232; email: alexander@doctors.org.uk.

Opioids and Pain Relief: A Historical Perspective,
Progress in Pain Research and Management, Vol.
25, edited by Marcia L. Meldrum, IASP Press,
Seattle, © 2003.

9

The Opiate Receptor: Scientific Treasure Trove

Marcia L. Meldrum

John C. Liebeskind History of Pain Collection, Louise M. Darling Biomedical Library, and Department of History, University of California, Los Angeles, Los Angeles, California, USA

In March 1973 a paper appeared in *Science* that opened many doors to the understanding of opiate drugs and how they worked in the human body. The authors, Candace Pert and Solomon Snyder of Johns Hopkins University, had identified "a component of nervous tissue" that could "selectively form complexes with opiate drugs at very low concentrations." They had identified sites on cellular membranes where particular molecules formed strong chemical bonds with opiate molecules so that the opiate substance "stuck" to the tissue. It was the first "direct demonstration" of the existence of a hypothetical entity—the opiate receptor (Pert and Snyder 1973).

The paper came at a crucial time in the field, soon after the Liebeskind laboratory's presentation of its finding of stimulation-produced analgesia (Akil, this volume) and at a time when a number of scientists, including Hans Kosterlitz, John Hughes, Avram Goldstein, Eric Simon, and Lars Terenius were investigating the possibility of endogenous opiate-like substances and cellular opiate receptors (Faull and Nicholson, this volume). Pert and Snyder's work attracted excited attention in both the scientific and popular press. Almost immediately there were professional rewards. After finishing her Ph.D. in 1975, Pert became a staff fellow with her own laboratory at the National Institute of Mental Health (NIMH). Snyder, already a full professor at Hopkins, was named Distinguished Service Professor in 1977 and, in 1980, became chair of the newly created Department of Neuroscience (Kanigel 1986). Both scientists have continued to work on the chemistry of neurotransmission and have maintained high public profiles through speaking and writing to scientific and lay audiences.

In 1978 the two had a very public falling-out when Snyder, Kosterlitz, and Hughes were honored with the Lasker Award in Basic Biomedical Research. Established by the philanthropist Mary Lasker, whose sponsorship of medical research dates back to the 1930s, in honor of her husband Albert, the Lasker is probably the most prestigious honor in American biomedical science, and very often foreshadows a Nobel Prize a few years later. Snyder received the award specifically for the opiate receptor work; Pert, who believed that her personal contribution had been as significant as his, was furious. Although she had been only a graduate student at the time, she saw her relationship to Snyder as similar to Hughes' relationship to Kosterlitz; if Hughes deserved recognition, so did she. Her exclusion from the Lasker she attributed either to sexism or to Snyder's minimizing of her contribution when he discussed the research privately with the scientific elite (Kanigel 1986; Pert 1997). (It should be noted here that it is not unheard of for junior colleagues such as Pert to receive prestigious awards; for example, in 1954 John Enders declined to accept the Nobel Prize unless his Fellows, Frederick Robbins and Thomas Weller, who had successfully cultured poliovirus in his laboratory, shared the award, and the Nobel Committee complied with his wishes.)

Pert "broke the rules" of the scientific community; she made her anger known, first in a letter to Mary Lasker and then in the public press. As she acknowledges, her actions cost her the professional support of her mentor, Snyder; of his mentor, the Nobel Laureate Julius Axelrod; and of many other senior colleagues. There is no clear consensus, however; Pert has also had her defenders. It is possible that the controversy cost Snyder—and Kosterlitz and Hughes—the Nobel (Kanigel 1986; Pert 1997). Whatever the merits of the case, both scientists were left somewhat tarnished. In any of the published accounts, notably Robert Kanigel's excellent study of scientific mentorship (1986), Snyder comes across as a little too ruthless, a little too ambitious; Pert as a little too emotional, a little too demanding.

In this brief account, I can hardly hope to improve on Kanigel's work or add further detail than Snyder (1989) and Pert (1997) have provided in their own books. What I will attempt to do, relying on these three sources, is to describe how this work fits into a particular model of "doing science" and how the receptor work fits into the overall intent of this book to better understand the history of opiates and pain.

The model of scientific work exemplified by Snyder and Pert in 1973 is very different from many of the projects described in this book: Kosterlitz and Hughes' pursuit of the endogenous opioids, or the Rice laboratory's painstaking research on the morphine molecule, or Houde's and Rogers' years of work on analgesic efficacy. These projects represent one kind of science: the steady and methodical pursuit of an important goal. Other projects are perhaps less methodical, yet are equally dedicated labors of love: Twycross's validation of the hospice treatment program, for example. But then there are the scientific treasure hunters, who sail over the horizon out of a clear blue sky, decipher the treasure map, and capture the golden prize.

To call Snyder and Pert treasure hunters is not to speak disparagingly of their scientific creativity or the quality of their work. A successful prospector in any field has to be very smart, very resourceful, and very skilled at reading the terrain. But modern science is a kind of free market economy; quite frequently, a particularly elusive idea or piece of knowledge, perhaps one that a number of researchers have been hunting for a long time, suddenly goes up in value. Once it looked just like ordinary currency; now clearly it is treasure trove. The experienced searchers stick to their strategies and rely on their knowledge of the terrain, but other hunters are on the trail now. In 1953 it was the structure of DNA. In 1972 it was the opiate receptor.

There were three reasons for the receptor's increased value at that time: political, scientific, and practical. The political motivator was the change in American government policy represented by the Comprehensive Drug Abuse Prevention and Control Act of 1970. The Nixon Administration had reacted vigorously to intense public concern over the spread of illicit drug use and dependence from the inner city to the middle-class suburb and the college campus, not to mention the army units in southeast Asia. New funds were available for treatment programs, for drug education, and (through NIMH) for research. Surely scientists could discover some chemical or physiological etiology for addiction, some metabolic malfunction in the nervous system that could be repaired.

The idea of a receptor for the opiate drugs, a cellular protein that recognized and bound to the chemistry of morphine or heroin "like the fit of a key in a lock" (Snyder 1989) had immediate appeal to the policy makers. (It was not, of course, a new idea: Paul Ehrlich had proposed the lock and key metaphor in the 1880s.) Such a mechanism could explain why respectable middle-class people could get "hooked" on drugs; research might then suggest a way of making the locks unworkable. In 1971, Snyder's laboratory at Johns Hopkins, along with laboratories at five other U.S. universities, received federal funding to establish research centers to study the mechanisms of drug addiction (Snyder 1989).

But the opiate receptor was also a hypothetical key to two promising and rapidly growing new disciplines in science: chemical pharmacology and neuroscience. Chemical pharmacology, developed as a field after World War II by Bernard Brodie and Julius Axelrod, studied drugs not as clinical experiments to be validated by trials and statistical analysis but as chemical molecules that interacted with other molecules in the body—if the chemical activity was clearly understood, then the effects of the drug, both positive and negative, ought to be clear as well (Kanigel 1986). At least, that was the theory. Demonstrating the existence of a cellular receptor that bound chemically to a well-known class of drugs would open up this field in a spectacular way.

The group of anatomists, physiologists, pharmacologists, psychologists, and biochemists whose interests coalesced around the brain and the nervous system—the Society for Neuroscience had been founded only the year before, in 1971—also found the idea of an opiate receptor appealing. The importance of neurotransmitter proteins in the rapid circulation of information through the central nervous system had become clear in the previous 20 years. But a system in which any neuron responded to any transmitter would be nothing but noise and chaos. Therefore, there had to be a chemical label or clue that enabled each neuron to respond selectively to transmitters that carried "relevant" information. A cellular receptor was the perfect such mechanism (Snyder 1989). Because opiate drugs were known to work on the central nervous system, identifying an opiate receptor in nerve cells would verify this hypothesis of neurotransmission and open up a whole new area of research.

The third reason why the opiate receptor became a prime target of research interest at this time was practical: sufficient evidence showed that such a receptor existed, although still entirely hypothetical and for an exogenous drug rather than an endogenous compound, and that a research investment in the search might well pay off. Much of this evidence had been accumulated from the years of analgesic research at the University of Virginia, the University of Michigan, and the National Institutes of Health (Acker, this volume; Rice, this volume). First, it was well known that very small doses of opiates relieved pain, but that a slight change in the chemical structure of an opiate drug could create a compound that was virtually inert. These qualities of high potency and sensitivity suggested the existence of very selective internal mechanisms that responded readily to the "right" drug, but not to the "wrong" one. Of particular significance was the opiates' stereospecificity: a drug that was in form the mirror image of a potent opiate often had no effect in the body at all. This finding suggested that the physiological response was based on the structural fit between drug and cell—again strong evidence of a receptor.

Finally, several opiate antagonists such as naloxone, the drug used by Huda Akil to block stimulation-produced analgesia (Akil, this volume), had been developed in the analgesic research work. Antagonists, chemically similar to the active drugs, were very effective in blocking analgesic activity and other opiate effects, even after the opiate had already been administered. The logical explanation was that the structure of an antagonist was also a good fit for the cellular receptors, thus displacing the opiates, but that the compound lacked an additional hypothetical component that stimulated cellular activity (Kanigel 1986; Snyder 1989).

So the opiate receptor, previously a minor conjecture, had begun to look like scientific treasure trove. Of course, it could also be a myth, a kind of scientific El Dorado. In the previous months, three specific cellular receptors had been identified: for acetylcholine, insulin, and nerve growth factor. But these were all endogenous compounds produced by the body, not drugs looking for a docking port. Still, by the early 1970s, at least three researchers were in the hunt, trying to show that an opiate receptor was present on animal cells: Avram Goldstein in San Francisco, Eric Simon in New York, and Lars Terenius in Uppsala, Sweden.

At Johns Hopkins, Snyder and his graduate student, Pert, discussed the problem at some point in the summer of 1972. He was 34, very young for a full professor, and had two young daughters; she was 26, married with a 5-year-old son. She had been in his laboratory for more than a year, working on acetylcholine, which she had taken over from another researcher and found unexciting.

Both agree that their interest in the opiate receptor developed sometime after 1971, when Snyder heard Goldstein give a talk on his thus-far unsuccessful experiments. Snyder was not part of the narcotics elite, the International Narcotics Research Club. "I hardly knew heroin from horseradish," he has commented, but he needed a new direction for Pert. Although the acetylcholine work was a solid project, leading to a "virtually guaranteed" Ph.D., she has written that she "remained profoundly unmoved"; Snyder recalls that she "set no world records for enthusiasm or experimental progress." As her mentor, he decided to reassign her. "I proposed to her the idea of the opiate receptor. Candace was ecstatic—a project of her very own. We set to work immediately" (Kanigel 1986; Snyder 1989; Pert 1997).

Pert agrees that she found the choline work uninspiring and distasteful. She remembers that, when Snyder brought up the Goldstein lecture over dinner at his home, the discussion was prompted after she described taking opiates for the pain of a serious injury, shortly before she came to Hopkins, and "the blissful state of consciousness" that resulted. She recalls that the idea of a quest for the opiate receptor held immediate strong appeal for her: "here was a goal I could easily imagine pursuing, a project worthy of my dreams … unraveling the mystery of how the opiates worked to produce their magical, otherworldly effects." Snyder, she has written, was "skeptical" and "ambivalent" when *she* approached *him* and asked to change her project, but agreed to let her try (Pert 1997). But she has also described how the project appealed to the ambition of both professor and student: "if I succeeded, then I just might become famous—as a graduate student who had actually done an exciting and original piece of work" (Pert 1997). "Sol had also recognized the possibility of scoring a coup, slipping in front of Avram [Goldstein] and waltzing away with the prize" (Pert 1997). So the team embarked on a treasure hunt.

Goldstein had provided a part of the map with his procedures, which he had described in the talk at Hopkins and later published (Goldstein 1971). The problem was to bind opiates to their receptors in vitro, in such a way that the bound drug could be measured, identified, or visualized. It was a difficult conundrum, because no one knew where the receptors were or to which part of the opiate molecule they attached themselves. The logical method to use was radioactive labeling, but even though this technique produced very clear results, there was the further problem of differentiating the receptor-bound drug from "nonspecific" binding—the drug would bind loosely to many molecules in any tissue, whether or not any target receptors were there.

Goldstein and his colleagues used radioactive levorphanol, a synthetic compound with a clearly understood structure. They mixed it with homogenized cell membranes from mouse brain and ran a count to see how much drug had been bound. The count was quite high due to a lot of nonspecific binding. Then they tried a mixture of radioactive and nonradioactive drug and ran another count. The working hypothesis was that the radioactivity would be lower in the second batch, because some of the receptor sites would be occupied with "hot" levorphanol and some with "cold." Then they mixed up a new batch of mouse brain and nonlabeled dextrorphan, the right-hand mirror-image isomer of levorphanol. The dextrorphan, they hoped, would saturate the membranes—except for the receptor sites, where it would not fit. Then they added the radioactive levorphanol and ran their final count.

Goldstein's hope was that the difference in counts between the first two experiments would give him a measure of overall nonspecific binding, that the difference between the second and the third would give him a measure of specific binding to opiate receptors, and that the comparison of all the counts would prove that the receptors were there. But the difference between the second two experiments was too low to be definitive. The nonradioactive levorphanol reduced the radioactive count (after the experiments had been repeated several times) by a little less than 2% more than the dextrorphan. So the opiate receptor might be there. Or it might not (Goldstein 1971; Kanigel 1986; Snyder 1989).

Snyder was fairly sure that he could improve on Goldstein's method by reducing the nonspecific binding. Both he and Pert seem to agree that he mapped the original experimental strategy. His first idea was to use a smaller amount of very "hot" drug as the experimental opiate; it was a safe assumption that the drug would have a high affinity for its own receptors and would bind preferentially to those sites. The second tactic was to use a filtration-and-wash method developed by Snyder's friend, Pedro Cuatrecasas, who had used it to demonstrate the existence of the insulin receptor, and then, in collaboration with Snyder's laboratory, to find the nerve growth factor receptor (Cuatrecasas 1972; Snyder 1989). As Pert has described the use of the rapid filtration machine, "the cellular soup would be sucked away with a strange *whhhhoooosssshhhhkkk* sound, leaving only the bound material stuck onto the receptor," and the washing process would rinse away any remaining loosely bound material. She spent some time learning to use the device, the Multiple Manifold Machine or "Triple-M" originally built for Marshall Nirenberg. Snyder ordered a supply of dihydromorphine labeled with tritium from New England Nuclear. Then they were ready to start (Snyder 1989; Pert 1997).

For several weeks, Pert mixed the "hot" dihydromorphine with rat organ tissue, mixed the control batches of levorphanol and dextrorphan, filtered, washed, and ran the counter. No matter how she varied her methods, the counts showed no consistent measurable difference, nothing that announced the presence of a receptor. Both she and Snyder became discouraged.

He has written: "Too much patience can be disastrous for a scientist. I have witnessed students immersing themselves for several years in dead-end projects. ... I was feeling sufficiently discouraged that dropping the opiate receptor work seemed the best choice. Candace, on the other hand, felt more inclined to give it another try. ... Perhaps receptors would be detectable only with antagonists." An opiate antagonist like naloxone would have to have a very high affinity to the receptors to be able to inhibit morphine, as it was known to do clinically. Naloxone, however, was only available by custom order. New England Nuclear "would label the naloxone with tritium and send it to us in a crude, unpurified state with no guarantees whatsoever. ... I agreed to accept the risks" (Snyder 1989).

In Pert's story, it was she who took the risk. "Sol called me into his office and told me he was going to shut down the opiate receptor assay. I was crushed. There were too many other things to do, he told me. ... In addition ... he was responsible for seeing that I got my Ph.D. ... it had been a long shot from the start ... and now I was expected to gracefully dive back into the original choline project." Pert had just finished reading an article about antagonist binding, however, and it gave her an idea. She knew where she could borrow some "cold" naloxone: from her husband Agu, an army chemical warfare researcher at Edgewood Arsenal. She sent it secretly to New England Nuclear to be labeled, purified it secretly, and quietly did the experiment, using naloxone, levorphanol, and dextrorphan, on a Friday afternoon after everyone else had left. Early on Monday, she recorded the radiation counts and found "a signal so loud it practically shrieked in my face. ... This was the killer experiment of my dreams, and I'd done it. I'd found the opiate receptor." According to her, Snyder was away that day at a conference (Pert 1997).

Whichever account is more accurate, the naloxone results thrilled both scientists. Snyder assigned his best technician, Adele Snowman, to work with Pert and see what other findings could be quickly gleaned. Endo Laboratories was now willing to donate quantities of naloxone, while Roche, Lilly, and Winthrop contributed the other drugs needed. Within a month, the team had demonstrated that the greatest number of opiate receptors was in brain cells, specifically in the corpus striatum, which showed twice as many as there were in the intestine. No receptors were found in the cerebellum or in human red blood cells. Once the binding sites were identified, Snyder and Pert were able to use them as an assay for different opiates, demonstrating that the pharmacological potency of methadone, codeine, and propoxyphene was directly proportional to their affinity to the receptors. They wrote their first report within weeks and submitted it to *Science* on December 1, 1972 (Pert and Snyder 1973; Snyder 1989).

Only a couple of months had passed since they had started the project. They had come into the game late; they had borrowed the pieces of the map from Goldstein and Cuatrecasas, but only Pert and Snyder had figured out how to read it correctly; they had sailed fast and straight past their fellows and found the gold.

Those who stake successful claim to a treasure sought by many are not always popular, especially when it is clear that their margin of victory is very slight. Goldstein wrote to Snyder noting gently that the paper in *Science* had been "a little ungenerous about the scientific and intellectual precedents of your work." Eric Simon, too, showed some ill feeling when an article Snyder wrote failed to recognize his earlier work on the problem (Snyder 1989). Lars Terenius might have been annoyed as well; he had demonstrated the higher inhibition of dihydromorphine binding to nerve endings by levomethadone than dextromethadone, a clear indication of specific opiate receptors, earlier in the year and sent his paper to *Acta Pharmacologica Toxicologica* in November. But the Scandinavian publication worked on a slower schedule and the paper did not appear until shortly after Pert and Snyder's had been published in March (Terenius 1973).

The crux of this story is the sudden salience of the opiate receptor in 1972. Many years of scientific work on analgesia, on pharmacology, on neurochemistry intersected with political and social interests at a specific time in history, and consequently a rather dubious hypothesis became worth proving. With another set of intersections—an ambitious scientist, the availability of a special technology, a student who did not follow the rules, a drug borrowed from an army arsenal—the hypothesis became a detectable reality.

Like opium itself, the idea of the opiate receptor was both attractive and alarming. It might offer clues and explanations to many problems, but one thing would be clear: whatever opiates do to the brain and the body, it is something the body has evolved to need and welcome. The finding of the receptor and, shortly after, of the endogenous opioids, opened the way to understand more about how we give ourselves (and respond to) both pleasure and pain; despite all the progress that neuroscience has made in the last 30 years, we are still wary about the implications of that knowledge. The most notable lesson to have emerged in humanity's long history with opium and its derivatives is recognizing how closely we all are bound to them.

REFERENCES

Cuatrecasas P. Isolation of the insulin receptor from liver and fat-cell membranes (detergent-solubilized-(125 I)insulin-polyethylene-glycol precipitation-sephadex). *Proc Natl Acad Sci USA* 1972; 69:318–322.

Goldstein A, Lowney LI, Pal BK. Stereospecific and nonspecific interactions of the morphine congener levorphanol in subcellular fractions of mouse brain. *Proc Natl Acad Sci USA* 1971; 68:1742–1747.

Kanigel R. *Apprentice to Genius: The Making of a Scientific Dynasty.* Baltimore: Johns Hopkins University Press, 1986.

Pert CB. *Molecules of Emotion: Why You Feel the Way You Feel.* New York: Simon and Schuster, 1997.

Pert CB, Snyder SH. The opiate receptor: demonstration in nervous tissue. *Science* 1973; 179:1011–1014.

Snyder SH. *Brainstorming: The Science and Politics of Opiate Research.* Cambridge, MA: Harvard University Press, 1989.

Terenius L. Stereospecific interaction between narcotic analgesics and a synaptic plasma membrane fraction of rat cerebral cortex. *Acta Pharmacol Toxicol (Copenhagen)* 1973; 32:317–320.

Correspondence to: Marcia L. Meldrum, PhD, Department of History, Bunche 6265, Box 951473, University of California, Los Angeles, Los Angeles, CA 90095-1473, USA. Email: meldrum@history.ucla.edu.

Opioids and Pain Relief: A Historical Perspective,
Progress in Pain Research and Management, Vol.
25, edited by Marcia L. Meldrum, IASP Press,
Seattle, © 2003.

10

History of the Development of Pain Management with Spinal Opioid and Non-Opioid Drugs

Michael J. Cousins

*Department of Anaesthesia and Pain Management, Royal North Shore
Hospital; Pain Management Research Institute, Royal North Shore Hospital
and University of Sydney, Sydney, New South Wales, Australia*

The long history of spinal administration of local anesthetics prompted the use of opioids by the spinal route. This chapter reviews the development of intrathecal and epidural administration and describes how technical expertise and a growing confidence in the advantages of potent spinal analgesia laid the groundwork for the early clinical use of spinal opioids. This advance occurred soon after the discovery of opioid receptors, endogenous opioids, and a spinal site of opioid action in animals.

DEVELOPMENT OF THE INTRATHECAL ROUTE

A New York neurologist, Leonard Corning, has been credited with the earliest attempt to use the spinal route for analgesia (see Brown and Fink 1998). It appears that he intended to deliver cocaine directly to the spinal cord, but apparently he was ignorant of the anatomy of the meninges and the cerebrospinal fluid. Corning placed his needle in the interspinous region at the T10–T11 level in the belief that blood vessels in the region would deliver the drug directly to the spinal cord. His technique involved a needle with a depth marker placed at the transverse process. In the low thoracic region, a drug so administered would probably be delivered into the epidural space rather than intrathecally. The credit for deliberately inserting a needle into the cerebrospinal fluid should go to Heinrich Quincke, who in 1891 used a lumbar puncture to treat hydrocephalus. Quincke's spinal needle technique was based on Wynter's use of Southey's tube for the treatment of spinal tuberculosis (Brown and Fink 1998).

August Bier in Germany and Theodore Tuffier in France independently administered local anesthetic (cocaine) into the cerebrospinal fluid in 1899 (Brown and Fink 1998). It is significant that even Tait and Caglieri, in their early writings of 1900, recognized that spinal administration of local anesthetics could cause neurotoxicity.

DEVELOPMENT OF THE EPIDURAL ROUTE

Interest in caudal epidural administration grew slowly but steadily in the first part of the 20th century (Brown and Fink 1998). In 1901, Cathelin and Sicard independently recognized the possibilities of this route. However, not until 1909 did Stoeckel describe the use of single-shot caudal epidural analgesia for obstetrical pain. Pages first reported the use of the lumbar epidural route for local anesthetics in 1921, and Dogliotti popularized its use for surgery in 1931. Building on the work of Stoeckel, Edwards and Hingson in 1942 described the first obstetrical use of continuous caudal analgesia. The worldwide adoption of epidural analgesia for labor pain quickly followed. In 1949, Curbelo introduced a technique for continuous epidural analgesia for surgery; his method was a key technical advance for the treatment of acute, chronic, and cancer pain.

The early 1950s and 1960s saw many leading anesthesiologists reporting case series and recommending epidural analgesia for pain relief in surgical and trauma patients. In his text *The Management of Pain* (1953), the founding father of the field of pain management, John J. Bonica, advocated the "top-up" method of epidural analgesia for postoperative pain relief. (This method uses intermittent doses injected by syringe via an indwelling epidural catheter.) Philip Bromage, another epidural pioneer, also promoted the top-up method following surgery and in trauma cases in his work *Spinal Epidural Analgesia* (1954). Simpson and his group in the United Kingdom used thoracic epidural catheters and top-up injections for a postoperative case series in 1961. They reported excellent pain relief and a reduction in respiratory complications with the method. Similarly, in 1965, Lloyd and colleagues found that patients receiving top-up thoracic epidural analgesia for the treatment of chest trauma showed unprecedented improvement in pain relief and other outcomes. Finally, in 1966, Green and Dawkins described the epidural use of a local anesthetic infusion to treat postoperative pain (Bryan-Brown 1986). In a graphic case report on the treatment of severe chest trauma, Bromage (1967) drew further attention to the potential benefits of epidural delivery in thoracic regional analgesia; his report helped stimulate clinicians to improve the treatment of post-trauma pain.

Despite these early opinions and reports of success from leaders in the field, the literature included little objective documentation of improved outcomes in postoperative or post-trauma pain following spinal epidural analgesia. All these early studies used local anesthetic alone, with the potential disadvantages of hypotension and motor dysfunction, i.e., "nonselective" neural blockade. More objective evidence of positive outcomes began to emerge in 1971 when Cousins and Wright reported that epidural analgesia with local anesthetic improved vascular graft blood flow in patients undergoing lower-limb vascular surgery. However, not until 1991 did Tuman and colleagues conclusively demonstrate that this technique could improve vascular graft outcomes.

Two papers in the 1980s provided further evidence for the benefits of postoperative epidural analgesia. Modig and colleagues (1981) reported a lower risk of thromboembolism in patients undergoing hip surgery, and Sheinin and colleagues (1987) described the reduced incidence of paralytic ileus in association with abdominal surgery. Nevertheless, not until 1998 did Ballantyne, Carr, and colleagues systematically review studies of epidural analgesia and its effects on respiratory complications. They concluded that this technique did indeed reduce respiratory complications. Throughout this period, Kehlet and colleagues made major contributions by focusing attention on effects of spinal analgesia on outcome, particularly postsurgical metabolism (see Kehlet and Wilmore 2002).

Finally, in 2002, a multicenter prospective study (the Master Trial) clearly documented a reduction in respiratory complications with administration of epidural local anesthetics (and in many cases opioids) to relieve postoperative pain (Rigg et al. 2002). Also in 2002, Barratt and colleagues reported that a multimodal analgesic regime, including epidural local anesthetics and opioids, was associated with the preservation of total body protein following major upper abdominal and thoracic surgery. Thus, after 30 years, strong evidence has borne out the early clinical observations of the 1970s indicating the benefits of the spinal route for acute pain relief.

SCIENTIFIC BASIS OF SPINAL OPIOIDS

SPINAL REFLEX ACTIVITY

While clinicians were exploring the epidural route, physiologists were observing the effects of spinal opiate drugs in animals. As long ago as 1937, Bodo and Brooks studied cats in which the spinal cord had been severed from the brain and documented that systemic administration of morphine reduced the spinal reflex activity induced by noxious (unpleasant or painful) stimuli. Interestingly, this research also showed that systemic morphine administration could reduce the increase in the animal's blood glucose normally associated with noxious stimuli. Experiments in spinalized dogs by Wikler and Frank (1948) showed that nociceptive reflex activity could be reduced by systemic morphine administration. Houde and colleagues (1951) reported comparative effects of opiates in the same preparation. These three studies were significant because the spinal preparation eliminated the influence of supraspinal mechanisms; thus, the action of systemic morphine on the spinal cord was the only possible cause of the reduction in polysynaptic nociceptive reflex activity at the spinal level.

The work of Hagbarth and Kerr (1954) suggesting that central influences impinged on spinal afferent activity was the true precursor of subsequent concepts of "descending modulation." The authors stimulated various regions of the brain, including the midbrain reticular formation, and found that supramaximal electrical stimulation of dorsal roots modified activity in dorsal columns. They postulated that descending central inputs may have inhibited sensory relays in the cord. Takagi and colleagues (1955) described the effects of opiate analgesics on spinal reflex activity, and Koll et al. (1963) reported that small intravenous doses of morphine reduced nociceptive reflexes in spinalized cats. All these findings suggested the potential of pain alleviation through the use of drugs that modified sensory transmission in the spinal cord.

ANALGESIC SYSTEMS

Possibly one of the earliest proposals for specific opioid receptors in the spinal cord arose from work on spinalized dogs by Martin and colleagues (1964). In a classic paper in the *Journal of Pharmacology and Experimental Therapeutics,* Martin clearly suggested a spinal action of opioids; subsequent publications built upon this proposal. A key step in establishing the presence of opioid receptors was the synthesis of naloxone by Fishman, and confirmation by Blumberg that it was an opioid antagonist. Their work appeared separately, first as an abstract in *Federation Proceedings* bearing Blumberg's name (Blumberg et al. 1961); not until 1966 was a patent for naloxone approved, bearing Fishman's name (Lewenstein and Fishman 1966).

The concept of delivering opiates directly to the neuraxis probably traces to the work of the Chinese scientists Tsou and Zhang, who in 1964 reported analgesia following microinjection of opiate into various brain areas, including the periaqueductal gray. However, Melzack and Wall gave the greatest conceptual impetus to other researchers with their paper on the gate control theory, proposing both spinal and supraspinal modulation of noxious input. Their theory received widespread attention following publication in *Science* in 1965.

Four years later, David Reynolds gave a major boost to the concept of analgesic systems dependent upon precisely located receptor areas. He reported that focal brain stimulation, particularly in the periaqueductal gray area, produced an analgesia in rats so profound that he was able to perform surgery without anesthetic (Reynolds 1969). John Liebeskind's laboratory in the late 1960s also studied rats to explore brain sites associated with pain. To their surprise, rats exhibited a reduced response to noxious stimulation following stimulation of the periaqueductal gray, among other sites (Liebeskind et al. 1973). The investigators coined a new term: "stimulation-produced analgesia" (SPA).

In a key paper in *Science,* one of Liebeskind's graduate students, David Mayer, reported that SPA resulted from periaqueductal gray stimulation and proposed the activation of some neural substrate that blocked transmission of the nociceptive stimulus (Mayer et al. 1971). Another research student, Huda Akil, working initially with nalorphine and then with naloxone, produced partial reversal of SPA by giving these opioid antagonists prior to stimulation. Her initial report (Akil et al. 1972) gave valuable assistance to Hans Kosterlitz and John Hughes in their hunt for endogenous opioid-like substances (see Akil, this volume).

At about this time, several laboratories followed the lead of Tsou and Zhang and further explored microinjection of opioids into the periaqueductal gray (Bradley and Dray 1973; Frederickson and Norris 1976). These varied studies suggested that SPA and the analgesia elicited by microinjection of morphine shared a common mechanism. Some researchers proposed that both morphine and endogenous opioids mimicked electrical stimulation by inhibiting the firing of tonically active inhibitory interneurons, but no direct evidence substantiated this hypothesis at that time. Nevertheless, the work of Mayer, Akil, Reynolds, and others provided a significant impetus to the concept of site-specific delivery of opioids.

The pivotal years were 1971–1973. Avram Goldstein suggested that the brain has stereospecific opioid receptors (see Akil, this volume). The assay he used did not provide conclusive evidence, but within 2 years, three independent groups identified the hypothesized receptors. Although Solomon Snyder and Candace Pert (1973) received the major credit with their report in *Science,* Lars Terenius (1973) and Eric Simon et al. (1973) provided equally important and independent corroboration. Terenius had performed the definitive work in 1972, but his publication was delayed until 1973 and appeared in a more obscure journal (Terenius 1973).

Finally, in a 1975 paper in *Nature*, Hughes, Smith, and Kosterlitz confirmed the existence of endogenous opioids. Thus, all the key pieces were in place suggesting the location of opioid receptors at specific sites throughout the neuraxis, some presumably located in the spinal cord, and acted upon by endogenous opioids. However, these studies presented no indication that spinal opioid receptors would have any significance for treatment of pain in humans.

SINGLE-CELL STUDIES

At the same time, electrophysiologists had begun to compile evidence by recording from single cells in the animal spinal cord after either systemic or direct electrophoretic injection of morphine. In one of the earliest studies, Jean-Marie Besson's group (1973) reduced normal dorsal horn responses to noxious stimuli by administering the opioid phenoperidine intravenously. In 1974, Kitahata and colleagues reported a similar reduction in neuronal firing in the cord after administering morphine intravenously to spinalized cats. The implication of these studies, although subsequently proved incorrect, was that morphine acted directly on spinal cord neurons in the deep dorsal horn (lamina V). In the same year, Calvillo and colleagues (1974) administered morphine in an area near dorsal horn cell bodies, heated the animal's skin to a normally painful level, and recorded measurable reduction in the normal excitation of dorsal horn neurons.

Duggan and colleagues conducted the definitive study 2 years later. They used electrophoretic injection of morphine in the superficial spinal cord dorsal horn, in the area called the substantia gelatinosa (SG), followed by electrophysiological recording of SG cell activity. Morphine administration in the SG selectively reduced the excitation of dorsal horn neurons in response to noxious heating of the skin, but showed relatively little effect on neuronal responses to hair deflection. The morphine action was long-lasting, but was reversed by naloxone, either when administered at the same spinal sites or when given intravenously in low doses (Duggan et al. 1976). In studies published in the same year, LeBars and colleagues (1976) and Jurna and Grossman (1976) reported similar reductions of neural activity in spinalized cats in response to painful stimuli.

PIVOTAL BASIC STUDIES

Duggan's work confirmed that morphine directly affected nociceptive activity in the dorsal horn of the spinal cord. However, the question of clinical application remained. Atweh and Kuhar (1977) used autoradiographic localization to confirm that the SG had the highest density of opioid receptors in the spinal cord.

Yaksh and Rudy (1976a) confirmed that intrathecal morphine administration produced dose-dependent, stereospecific, naloxone-reversible analgesia in rats. When this key study was first submitted to *Science*, the work of Atweh and Kuhar had not yet been published, and the paper by Duggan and colleagues was under review by the editors of *Nature*. The *Science* reviewers doubted the strength of the evidence that opioid receptors in the spinal cord were capable of producing spinally mediated analgesia. Yaksh and Rudy defended their conclusions vigorously, and the paper was accepted for publication. Soon after, Jessel and Iversen (1977) reported that opioids inhibit the release of substance P, a key neurotransmitter of noxious information, from the trigeminal nucleus, and Zieglgansberger and Bayer (1976) reported that morphine reduced the postsynaptic excitation of SG neurons evoked by glutamate. These papers confirmed the role of spinal opioid receptors in modifying spinal transmission of noxious input.

The series of studies by Yaksh and Rudy (1976a,b, 1977) depended significantly on their previously developed techniques for inserting a permanent spinal catheter and administering intrathecal drugs in rat, rabbit, cat, and primate models. This method permitted them to document numerous effects, including long-lasting elevation of nociceptive threshold; decreased thermal, mechanical, and visceral responses; analgesic effects involving subpopulations of opioid receptors; and selective effects on pain behavior in the absence of motor function effects. Their additional detailed studies in animals provided information concerning dose response, potencies, receptor systems, mechanisms of analgesia, neurotoxicity, development of tolerance, and interactions between opioid- and non-opioid-mediated effects. Subsequently, researchers synthesized selective opioid ligands and identified several anti-opioid systems involving substance P, cholecystokinin, excitatory amino acids, protein kinase C, and nitric oxide. Yaksh and others administered spinal opioids and non-opioids and studied their effects in various neuropathic models.

CLINICAL RESEARCH

The studies in spinalized animals paralleled early spinal opioid work with patients. In March 1979, Willer began studies of morphine administered intravenously to paraplegic patients and recorded reduced spinal polysynaptic reflex activity that would normally have been evoked by nociceptive stimulation of the sural nerve of the calf. Willer and Bussel's publication in 1980 implied that the systemic morphine had produced a direct effect on the spinal cord, because the patients' paraplegia precluded descending influences from the brain. The effects were reversible by naloxone, and monosynaptic activity was not affected. It is clear that Willer was thinking about the clinical potential of spinal opioids. It is surprising, however, given the inadequacy of systemic methods of opioid administration for the treatment of acute, chronic, and cancer pain, that clinicians had not moved to this option sooner.

As early as 1975, the research group that Laurence Mather and I led in Adelaide, Australia, had begun studying the pharmacokinetics and pharmacodynamics of opioid drugs administered to patients by various routes. We planned to examine all routes of administration, but our initial studies focused on intravenous, intramuscular, and oral routes, a first priority given the lack of a proper scientific basis for these methods of clinical opioid administration. As Duggan's laboratory was close by in Canberra, our group soon learned of his work on the SG (Duggan et al. 1976). Peter Wilson, a member of our team in 1975, moved on to work with Yaksh at the Mayo Clinic and published a paper on analgesic effects of intrathecal baclofen (Wilson and Yaksh 1978), and then returned to work with us.

Nevertheless, Mather and I had significant concerns about the potential neurotoxicity of opioids administered via the spinal route. We were spurred on, however, by the papers of Snyder and Pert (1973) and Hughes et al. (1975), and in particular by a paper by Akil et al. (1976) in *Science,* which suggested (as had Yaksh and Rudy's first report) that the lumbar spinal administration of opioids may have a powerful direct effect on the spinal cord and possibly also on key brain sites such as the periaqueductal gray. Our group prepared an application to the Institutional Human Ethics Committee to enable us to proceed with integrated studies of the pharmacokinetics and pharmacodynamics of spinally administered opioids, but the significant lack of neurotoxicity data delayed approval for such studies.

At the Mayo Clinic, neurosurgeon Fred Kerr, head of Tony Yaksh's department and a council member of the International Association for the Study of Pain (IASP), strongly encouraged researchers to move into clinical studies. Kerr guided the submission to the Human Ethics Committee, which allowed Wang and colleagues (1979) to conduct a case series of studies of intrathecal morphine administration in humans. Shortly thereafter, Behar and his colleagues in Israel (1979) reported a clinical case series of epidural morphine administration, with anecdotal evidence of pain reductions in several types of human pain states.

By 1979, our research group in Adelaide had made good advances with our systematic studies of epidural and intrathecal opioids, and we were impressed by the initial pharmacokinetic data. In a letter to the *Lancet* (Cousins et al. 1979), we presented cerebrospinal fluid and blood kinetic data that strongly suggested a spinal site of action for epidurally administered meperidine. We also reported parallel information about analgesic response and the lack of effects on sympathetic and motor function. These observations and findings prompted us to suggest the term "selective spinal analgesia." The proposed terminology led to substantial debate in the letters section of the *Lancet*. The concept of selective spinal analgesia encapsulated researchers' continuing attempts to produce analgesia with optimal efficacy, but without the effects on motor function and blood pressure associated with spinal administration of local anesthetics.

In the same year, two reports of delayed respiratory depression in cancer patients following intrathecal administration of morphine appeared in the same volume of the *Lancet*, one from the Adelaide group (Glynn et al. 1979; Liolios and Anderson 1979). Shortly thereafter, Davies et al. (1980) and Boas (1980) published corroborating reports. There followed a virtual explosion of uncontrolled anecdotal clinical reports, few of which added new knowledge regarding spinal administration of opioids (see Cousins and Mather 1984). Torda and colleagues (1980) used a rigorous "Latin square" design to conduct the first controlled study comparing intramuscular with epidural morphine. The full account of our group's integrated spinal opioid pharmacokinetic and pharmacodynamic study then appeared in *Anesthesiology* (Glynn et al. 1981).

Anesthesiologists remained concerned about the mechanisms of delayed respiratory depression involved in spinal opioid administration and the potential hazard to patients. In 1982, Bromage and colleagues documented changes in carbon dioxide response in a group of volunteers. The response paralleled clinical evaluation of analgesic spread, a finding that suggested the progressive migration of opioid in the cerebrospinal fluid (CSF) toward brainstem respiratory centers. In 1983, Nordberg and colleagues reported peak morphine concentrations in the CSF about 40–90 minutes after lumbar epidural administration.

To address the issue of possible brain effects of spinally administered opioids, the Adelaide group systematically evaluated the cephalad migration of morphine from the lumbar region to the cervical CSF; our papers documented that on average morphine peaked in the cervical CSF approximately 180 minutes after lumbar administration (Gourlay et al. 1985, 1987). Lipophilicity emerged as an important factor in our studies that compared the cephalad migration of morphine with pethidine, fentanyl, and hydromorphone (Gourlay et al. 1985, 1987; Brose et al. 1991). In 1989, Gustafsson used [11]C (radiolabeled) morphine to confirm that morphine migrates from lumbar to cervical levels after about 170 minutes.

Finally, a major nationwide study in Sweden documented that, with appropriate minimal clinically effective doses, the incidence of respiratory events associated with spinal administration of morphine differed little from that following intramuscular administration (Rawal et al. 1987). With the scientific insights gleaned from these crucial CSF pharmacokinetic data and outcome studies, clinicians were at last able to proceed with safe and effective use of spinal opioids.

Although technically it cannot be described as spinal analgesia, intracerebroventricular (i.c.v.) administration of opioids is also a method of "site-directed" opioid delivery. Supraspinal activation of descending inhibitory pathways, which modulate activity in spinal dorsal horn, is the probable mediator in analgesia by this route, most likely via spinal serotonin receptor activation and associated release of the inhibitory neurotransmitter γ-aminobutyric acid (GABA) (Kawamata et al. 2002). Intracerebroventricular opioid administration was initially developed as a theoretically advantageous delivery site close to the nociception site in head and neck cancer (Leavens et al. 1982; Lenzi et al. 1985). However, several researchers soon found that i.c.v. administration also relieved cancer pain in upper and lower body regions (Nurchi 1984; Obbens et al. 1987; Cramond and Stuart 1993). Comparative data provided by Ballantyne and colleagues (1996) indicate that in patients with cancer pain, spinal epidural and intrathecal routes provide a level of analgesic efficacy similar to that obtained with i.c.v. administration.

LITERATURE REVIEWS

Several review papers on spinal opioid analgesia appeared in the early 1980s. Yaksh (1981) published a major review of the method's characteristics and principles of action, focusing on the basic science, but also presenting the modest amount of clinical information then available. In 1984, Duggan and North published a major review of opioid electrophysiology at both brain and spinal sites of action, and Cousins and Mather (1984) published an extensive review of intrathecal and epidural administration, focusing on the basic science and clinical evidence for the effects, side effects, and therapeutic index of this new option for the relief of acute, chronic, and cancer pain.

In a systematic evaluation of the entire pain literature, Strassels and colleagues (1999) reviewed more than 110,000 articles published between 1981 and 1997. The review by Cousins and Mather (1984) proved to be the fifth most frequently cited article and that by Yaksh (1981) ranked ninth; Yaksh was also second on the list of most frequently cited authors for his basic research papers on spinal opioid and non-opioid analgesia. These statistics are telling measures of the impact of spinal opioid analgesia on the field. In recent years, emphasis has shifted from opioid monotherapy to "spinal combination drug therapy." Carr and Cousins reviewed all the options in their 1988 book chapter on the spinal route of analgesia. In 1999, Dougherty and Staats reviewed the mechanisms and clinical evidence for intrathecal drug therapy for chronic pain. Most recently, Walker et al. (2002) systematically reviewed combination spinal opioid and non-opioid analgesia for acute, chronic, and cancer pain.

In conclusion, it is clear that the early basic and clinical studies of the spinal administration of opioids have stimulated intensive research on both the mechanisms and the method. The spinal cord has emerged as a major target for pain control, with the emphasis now on combination opioid and non-opioid analgesia. Since the early studies in the mid-1970s, much interest has focused on the key role played by spinal and supraspinal sensitization in the development of persistent pain. In the future, the spinal route of analgesia may be used to target spinal neuroplasticity changes, with the aim of preventing or treating pathophysiology associated with the development of persistent pain. The recent review by Walker et al. (2002) has suggested the new terminology "combination spinal analgesic chemotherapy" to describe this deliberate targeting strategy. As was the case at the first administration of a spinal opioid, the major concern and limitation of future development remains the availability of adequate neurotoxicity data.

REFERENCES

Akil H, Mayer DJ, Liebeskind JC. Comparaison chez le rat entre l'analgésie induite par stimulation de la substance grise peri-aqueductale et l'analgésie morphine. *CR Acad Sci (Paris)* 1972; 274:3603–3605.

Akil H, Mayer DJ, Liebeskind JC. Antagonism of stimulation produced analgesia by naloxone, a narcotic antagonist. *Science* 1976; 191:961–962.

Atweh SF, Kuhar MJ. Autoradiographic localization of opiate receptors in rat brain. I. Spinal cord and lower medulla. *Brain Res* 1977; 124:53–67.

Ballantyne JC, Carr DB, Berkey CS, et al. Comparative efficacy of epidural, subarachnoid, and intracerebroventricular opioids in patients with pain due to cancer. *Reg Anesth* 1996; 21:542–556.

Ballantyne JC, Carr DB, DeFerranti S, et al. The comparative effects of postoperative analgesic therapies on pulmonary outcome: cumulative meta-analyses of randomized, controlled trials. *Anesth Analg* 1998; 86:598–612.

Barratt SM, Smith RC, Kee AJ, Cousins MJ. Multimodal analgesia and intravenous nutrition preserves total body protein following major upper gastrointestinal surgery. *Reg Anesth Pain Med* 2002; 15:15–22.

Behar M, Olshwang D, Magora F, Davidson JT. Epidural morphine in treatment of pain. *Lancet* 1979; 1:527–529.

Besson JM, Wyon-Maillard MC, Benoist JM, Conseiller C, Hamann KF. Effects of phenoperidine on lamina V cells in the cat dorsal horn. *J Pharmacol Exp Ther* 1973; 187:239–245.

Blumberg H, Dayton HB, George M, Rapaport DN. N-allylnoroxymorphone: a potent narcotic antagonist. *Fed Proc* 1961; 20:311.

Boas RA. Hazards of epidural morphine. *Anaesth Intensive Care* 1980; 8:377–378.

Bodo RC, Brooks JMC. Effects of morphine on blood sugar and reflex activity in the chronic spinal cat. *Pharmacol Exp Ther* 1937; 61:82–88.

Bonica JJ. *The Management of Pain,* 1st ed. Philadelphia: Lea & Febiger, 1953.

Bradley PB, Dray A. Actions and interactions on microiontophoretically applied morphine with transmitter substances on brain stem neurones. *Br J Pharmacol* 1973; 47:642.

Bromage PR. *Spinal Epidural Analgesia.* Edinburgh: Livingstone, 1954.

Bromage PR. Extradural analgesia for pain relief. *Br J Anaesth* 1967; 39:721–729.

Bromage PR, Camporesi EM, Durant PA, Nielsen CH. Rostral spread of epidural morphine. *Anesthesiology* 1982; 56:431.

Brose WG, Tanelian DL, Brodsky JB, Mark JB, Cousins MJ. CSF and blood pharmacokinetics of hydromorphone and morphine following lumbar epidural administration. *Pain* 1991; 45:11–15.

Brown DL, Fink R. The history of neural blockade and pain management. In: Cousins MJ, Bridenbaugh PO (Eds). *Neural Blockade in Clinical Anesthesia and Pain Management,* 3rd ed. Philadelphia: Lippincott, 1998, pp 3–34.

Bryan-Brown C. Development of pain management in critical care. In: Cousins MJ, Phillips GD (Eds). *Acute Pain Management: Clinics in Critical Care Medicine.* New York: Churchill Livingstone, 1986, pp 1–19.

Calvillo O, Henry JL, Neuman RS. Effects of morphine and naloxone on dorsal horn neurones in the cat. *Can J Physiol Pharm* 1974; 61:82–88.

Carr DB, Cousins MJ. Spinal route of analgesia: opioids and future options. In: Cousins MJ, Bridenbaugh PO (Eds). *Neural Blockade in Clinical Anesthesia and Pain Management,* 3rd ed. Philadelphia: Lippincott, 1998, pp 915–983.

Cousins MJ, Mather LE. Intrathecal and epidural administration of opioids. *Anesthesiology* 1984; 61:276–310.

Cousins MJ, Wright CJ. Graft, muscle, skin blood flow after epidural block in vascular surgical procedures. *Surg Gynecol Obstet* 1971; 133:59–64.

Cousins MJ. Mather LE, Glynn CJ, Wilson PR, Graham JR. Selective spinal analgesia. *Lancet* 1979; 1:1141–1142.

Cramond T, Stuart G. Intraventricular morphine for intractable pain of advanced cancer. *J Pain Symptom Manage* 1993; 8:465–473.

Davies GK, Tolhurst-Cleaver CL, James TL. CNS depression from intrathecal morphine. *Anesthesiology* 1980; 52:280.

Dougherty PM, Staats PS. Intrathecal drug therapy for chronic pain. *Anesthesiology* 1999; 91:1891–1918.

Duggan AW, North RA. Electrophysiology of opioids. *Pharm Rev* 1984; 35:219–281.

Duggan AW, Hall JG, Headley PM. Morphine, enkephalin and the substantia gelatinosa. *Nature* 1976; 264:456–458.

Frederickson RCA, Norris FH. Enkephalin-induced depression of single neurons in brain areas with opiate receptors—antagonism by naloxone. *Science* 1976; 194:440–442.

Glynn CJ, Mather LE, Cousins MJ, Wilson PR, Graham JR. Spinal narcotics and respiratory depression. *Lancet* 1979; 2:356–357.

Glynn CJ, Mather LE, Cousins MJ, Graham JR, Wilson PR. Peridural meperidine in humans: analgetic response, pharmacokinetics, and transmission into CSF. *Anesthesiology* 1981; 55:520–526.

Gourlay GK, Cherry DA, Cousins MJ. Cephalad migration of morphine in CSF following lumbar epidural administration in patients with cancer pain. *Pain* 1985; 23:317–326.

Gourlay GK, Cherry DA, Plummer JL, Armstrong PJ, Cousins MJ. The influence of drug polarity on the absorption of opioid drugs into CSF and subsequent cephalad migration following lumbar epidural administration: application to morphine and pethidine. *Pain* 1987; 31:297–305.

Green R, Dawkins CJM. Postoperative analgesia: the use of continuous epidural block. *Anaesthesia* 1966; 21:322.

Gustafsson LL, Hartvig P, Bergstrom K, et al. Distribution of 11C-labelled morphine and pethidine after spinal administration to Rhesus monkey. *Acta Anaesthiol Scand* 1989; 33:105–111.

Hagbarth KE, Kerr DIB. Central influences on spinal afferent conduction. *J Neurophysiol* 1954; 17:295.

Houde RW, Wikler A, Irwin S. Comparative actions of analgesics, hypnotics and paralytic agents in hindlimb reflexes in chronic spinal dogs. *J Pharmacol Exper Ther* 1951; 103:243–248.

Hughes J, Smith IW, Kosterlitz HW, et al. Identification of two related pentapeptides from the brain with potent opiate agonist activity. *Nature* 1975; 258:577–579.

Jessel TM, Iversen LL. Opiate analgesics inhibit substance P release from rat trigeminal nucleus. *Nature* 1977; 268:549–551.

Jurna I, Grossman W. The effect of morphine on the activity evoked in ventrolateral tract axons of the cat spinal cord. *Exp Brain Res* 1976; 24:473–484.

Kawamata T, Omote K, Toriyabe M, et al. Intracerebroventricular morphine produces antinociception by evoking gamma-aminobutyric acid release through activation of 5-hydroxytryptamine 3 receptors in the spinal cord. *Anesthesiology* 2002; 95:1175–1182.

Kehlet H, Wilmore DW. Multimodal strategies to improve surgical outcome. *Am J Surg* 2002; 183:630–641.

Kitahata LM, Kosaka Y, Taub A, et al. Lamina specific suppression of dorsal horn unit activity by morphine sulfate. *Anesthesiology* 1974; 41:39–48.

Koll W, Haase J, Block G, Muhlberg B. The predilective action of small doses of morphine on nociceptive spinal reflexes of low spinal cats. *Int J Neuropharmacol* 1963; 2:57–65.

Leavens ME, Stratton Hill C, Cech DA, et al. Intrathecal and intraventricular morphine for pain in cancer patients: initial study. *J Neurosurg* 1982; 56:241–245.

LeBars D, Guilbaud D, Jurna I, Besson JM. Differential effects of morphine on responses of dorsal horn lamina V type cells elicited by A and C fibre stimulation in the spinal cat. *Brain Res* 1976; 115:518–524.

Lenzi A, Galli G, Gandolfini M, Marini G. Intraventricular morphine in proneoplastic painful syndrome of the cervicofacial region: experience in thirty eight cases. *Neurosurgery* 1985; 17:6–11.

Lewenstein MJ, Fishman J. Morphine derivative. U.S. patent 3.254.088, May 1966.

Liebeskind JC, Guilbaud G, Besson JM, Oliveras JL. Analgesia from electrical stimulation of the periaqueductal gray matter in the cat: behavioral observations and inhibitory effects on spinal cord interneurons. *Brain Res* 1973; 50:441–446.

Liolios A, Andersen FH. Selective spinal analgesia. *Lancet* 1979; 2:357.

Lloyd JW, Crampton-Smith A, O'Connor BT. Classification of chest injuries as an aid to treatment. *BMJ* 1965; 1:1518.

Martin WR, Eades CG, Fraser HF, Wikler A. Use of hindlimb reflexes of the chronic spinal dog for comparing analgesics. *J Pharmacol Exp Ther* 1964; 144:8–11.

Mayer DJ, Wolfe TL, Akil H, et al. Analgesia from electrical stimulation in the brainstem of the rat. *Science* 1971; 114:1351–1354.

Melzack R, Wall PD. Pain mechanisms: a new theory. *Science* 1965; 150:971.

Modig J, Hjelmstedt A, Sahlstedt B, Maripuu E. Comparative influences of epidural and general anaesthesia on deep venous thrombosis and pulmonary embolism after total hip replacement. *Acta Chir Scand* 1981; 147:125–130.

Nordberg G, Hedner T, Mellstrand T, Dahlstrom B. Pharmacokinetic aspects of epidural morphine analgesia. *Anesthesiology* 1983; 58:545–551.

Nurchi GN. Use of intraventricular and intrathecal morphine in intractable pain associated with cancer. *Neurosurgery* 1984; 15:801–803.

Obbens EA, Stratton Hill C, Leavens ME, et al. Intraventricular morphine administration for control of chronic cancer pain. *Pain* 1987; 28:61–68.

Rawal N, Amer S, Gustaffson LL, Allvin R. Present state of extradural and intrathecal opioid analgesia in Sweden: a nationwide follow up survey. *Br J Anaesth* 1987; 59:791.

Reynolds DV. Surgery in the rat during electrical analgesia induced by focal brain stimulation. *Science* 1969; 164:444.

Rigg JR, Jamrozik K, Myles PS, et al. Epidural anaesthesia and analgesia and outcome of major surgery: a randomized trial. *Lancet* 2002; 359:1276–1282.

Sheinin B, Asantila R, Orko R. The effect of bupivacaine and morphine on pain and bowel function after colonic surgery. *Acta Anaesthesiol Scand* 1987; 31:161–164.

Simpson BRJ, Parkhouse J, Marshall R, et al. Extradural analgesia and the prevention of postoperative respiratory complications. *Br J Anaesth* 1961; 33:628.

Simon EJ, Hiller JM, Edelman I. Stereospecific binding of the potent narcotic analgesic (3H) etorphine to rat brain homogenate. *Proc Natl Acad Sci USA* 1973; 70:1947–1949.

Snyder SH, Pert CB. Opiate receptor: demonstration in nervous tissue. *Science* 1973; 179:1011–1014.

Strassels SA, Carr DB, Meldrum M, Cousins MJ. Toward a canon of the pain and analgesia literature: a citation analysis. *Anesth Analg* 1999; 89:1528–1533.

Tait D, Caglieri G. Experimental and clinical notes on the subarachnoid space. *JAMA* 1900; 3516.

Takagi H, Matsumara M, Yanai A, Agiu K. The effect of analgesics on the spinal reflex activity of the cat. *Jpn J Pharmacol* 1955; 4:176–187.

Terenius L. Characteristics of the 'receptor' for narcotic analgesics in synaptic plasma membrane fraction from rat brain. *Acta Pharmacol Toxicol* 1973; 33:377–384.

Torda TA, Pybus DA, Liberman H, Clark M, Crawford M. Experimental comparison of extradural and IM morphine. *Br J Anaesth* 1980; 52:939–943.

Tsou K, Zhang CS. Studies on the site of analgesic action of morphine by intracerebral micro-injection. *Scientia Sinica* 1964; 13:1099–1109.

Tuman KJ, McCarthy RJ, March RJ, et al. Effects of epidural anesthesia and analgesia on coagulation and outcome after major vascular surgery. *Anesth Analg* 1991; 73:696–704.

Walker SM, Goudas LC, Cousins MJ, Carr DB. Combination spinal analgesic chemotherapy: a systematic review. *Anesth Analg* 2002; 95:674–715.

Wang JW, Nauss LA, Thomas JE. Pain relief by intrathecally applied morphine in man. *Anesthesiology* 1979; 50:149–151.

Wikler A, Frank J. Hindlimb reflexes of chronic spinal dogs during cycles of addiction to morphine and methadone. *J Pharmacol Exp Ther* 1948; 94:382–400.

Willer JC, Bussel B. Evidence for a direct spinal mechanism in morphine-induced inhibition of nociceptive reflexes in humans. *Brain Res* 1980; 187:212–215.

Wilson PR, Yaksh TL. Baclofen is antinociceptive in the spinal intrathecal space of animals. *Eur J Pharmacol* 1978; 51:323.

Yaksh TL. Spinal opiate analgesia: characteristics and principles of action. *Pain* 1981; 11:293–346.

Yaksh TL, Rudy TA. Analgesia mediated by a direct spinal action of narcotics. *Science* 1976a; 192:1357.

Yaksh TL, Rudy TA. Chronic catheterization of the spinal subarachnoid space. *Physiol Behav* 1976b; 17:1031–1036.

Yaksh TL, Rudy TA. Studies on the direct spinal action of narcotics in the production of analgesia in the rat. *J Pharmacol Exp Ther* 1977; 202:411–418.

Zieglgansberger W, Bayer H. The mechanisms of inhibition of neuronal activity by opiates in the spinal cord of the cat. *Brain Res* 1976; 115:111–128.

Correspondence to: Michael J. Cousins, MD, FFPMANZCA, FANZCA, FRCA, Department of Anesthesia and Pain Management, Royal North Shore Hospital, St. Leonards, NSW 2065, Australia. Email: mcousins@doh.health.nsw.gov.au.

Opioids and Pain Relief: A Historical Perspective,
Progress in Pain Research and Management, Vol.
25, edited by Marcia L. Meldrum, IASP Press,
Seattle, © 2003.

11

The World Health Organization Cancer Pain Relief Program

Mark Swerdlow

Late of Altrincham, Cheshire, United Kingdom

In 1981, Jan Stjernswärd, a Swedish oncologist, was newly appointed as head of the cancer unit of the World Health Organization (WHO). He decided to set up a three-pronged program of work for the unit: prevention (by eliminating cancer-promoting habits such as smoking and betel nut chewing), early detection and treatment, and relief of pain. This was the first time that WHO had concerned itself with any type of pain therapy. Stjernswärd required some advice on the management of cancer pain, and early in 1981 I was invited to undertake a consultancy with the WHO cancer unit for this purpose. I was an anesthetist and specialist in nerve blocks for pain relief of chronic pain, as well as cancer pain, at Hope Hospital, Salford, United Kingdom.

Stjernswärd and I felt that, because it was not possible to provide complete cancer treatment worldwide, we should at least endeavor to alleviate the patients' pain, as we wrote in 1982, for the "millions of sufferers ... who have no hope of cure and little chance of adequate relief from pain" (Swerdlow and Stjernswärd 1982). We planned to start by gathering data from countries in different parts of the world on the incidence of cancer and on the availability and effectiveness of various treatments.

We were well aware that the management of cancer pain worldwide was far from satisfactory at that time. A number of journalists and physicians had presented data on the suffering of cancer patients. John Bonica, founder and past president of the International Association for the Study of Pain (IASP), had gathered statistics from England, Italy, and the United States, which he presented at the First World Congress on Pain in 1975 and again at the First International Symposium on the Pain of Advanced Cancer in 1978. His figures indicated that 50–85% of advanced cancer patients suffered pain, often inadequately relieved (Bonica 1979).

During the year that we gathered data, Stjernswärd and I confirmed these estimates from our own observations, although we also found that traditional approaches were providing some relief in certain parts of the world. On a visit to a cancer hospital in Sri Lanka, I visited a women's ward that housed a large number of patients with advanced cancer, who appeared to be placid and not in pain; I was told that their sole medicament was aspirin. When I asked whether these patients were receiving any traditional medication, the doctor in charge replied that they were receiving Ayurvedic medicine, but he did not know the active constituents of the herbs administered. In Japan, under similar circumstances, I was told that acupuncture accounted for the apparent lack of suffering. In other areas, pain therapies were available only in urban centers. In responses to WHO questionnaires, Dr. Bernal from Panama stated: "If they can't go [to health centers], they get no treatment," and Dr. Martelete, whom Stjernswärd visited in Porto Alegre, Brazil, wrote: "They can't get narcotics except in hospitals. ... At home with cancer, nobody looks after them" (Swerdlow 1981).

Stjernswärd and I drew up a questionnaire and sent out 250 copies in March 1982 to doctors we had contacted previously in selected cancer clinics in 11 different countries (these included Nigeria, Egypt, Turkey, the Philippines, the Sudan, and Sweden); we requested that they return the completed questionnaires by September 1982. We also decided to bring together a small group of experts to discuss and help devise "a simple, practical scheme" of treatment. We therefore set about recruiting the expert cooperation of John Bonica, as well as Kathleen Foley of Memorial-Sloan-Kettering Cancer Center, New York; Vittorio Ventafridda of the National Cancer Institute, Milan; Robert Twycross of Sobell House, Oxford; and Anders Rane of Huddinge University Hospital, Stockholm. At this stage we started to make arrangements for a WHO consultation meeting, to be held at the beautiful 16th-century Villa d'Este on Lake Como, outside Milan, on October 14–15, 1982. With Ventafridda's help, we were able to obtain support for the meeting from the Floriani Foundation.

By September only five countries (Brazil, India, Israel, Japan, and Sri Lanka) had returned completed questionnaires, reporting data on 919 cancer patients. The data showed that only 10% of the patients reported complete pain relief from the treatment they were receiving and that more than a quarter of those who experienced severe pain (29%) reported little or no relief. Although the sample of patients was not statistically adequate, the results made it clear to all concerned that cancer pain was not being properly managed. Physicians from the five participating countries were invited to take part in the Milan meeting, but only four were able to attend: Jesmond Birkhan of Haifa, Israel; Fumikazu Takeda of Saitama, Japan; P.B. Desai, of Bombay, India; and Miriam Martelete of Brazil.

Prior to the Milan meeting, Stjernswärd and I drafted a paper on the problems of cancer pain that was published in the *World Health Forum* (Swerdlow and Stjernswärd 1982). This paper was translated into several languages and widely distributed with the result that our ideas regarding cancer pain relief reached a wide audience among the medical profession.

At the Milan consultation, participants explored in detail the reasons why cancer pain was so poorly managed and provided valuable advice on the most appropriate therapies to be recommended. The subject of cancer pain was at that time inadequately covered both in medical school curricula and in cancer textbooks. Ignorance and incorrect ideas about the nature of cancer pain, together with anxiety about the use of narcotic drugs and fear of the dangers of addiction, meant that patients were concerned about taking too much medication and doctors and nurses were often afraid of giving too much. All those present realized that any treatment measures they formulated at the meeting must be simple and readily applicable in developing countries as well as in more advanced nations, a policy that mandated the use of basic and readily available drugs. The therapy advocated would be a simple drug regimen that could be disseminated rapidly and cheaply even to the most remote villages in the developing world. The introduction of this model, which included the use of strong narcotic drugs, would require educating not only doctors and nurses but also national ministries of health.

As a result of the meeting, we prepared a draft set of guidelines that introduced the concept of the "three-step analgesic ladder" (Fig. 1). The recommended principles of treatment were as follows: Oral medication should be used as long as possible because it can be administered at home, allowing the patient to retain freedom of activity. The analgesic drugs should be given on a regular basis by the clock (*not* "as required"), and the dose should be titrated for the individual patient. In addition to analgesic drugs, the experts recommended the use of five different types of adjuvants to enhance analgesia and to treat attendant physical and psychological malaise. When cancer pain becomes persistent, the cause should be identified if possible and treated by radiotherapy, chemotherapy, or palliative surgery. To a large extent, the WHO cancer pain relief program was based on the pain management program developed by Cicely Saunders at St. Christopher's Hospice in London, and later

3. Strong opioid ± non-opioid ± adjuvant

2. Weak opioid ± non-opioid ± adjuvant

1. Non-opioid ± adjuvant

Fig. 1. The WHO three-step analgesic ladder for cancer pain treatment.

modified by Robert Twycross, based on the findings from his research there (for details see Faull and Nicholson, this volume).

Following the Milan consultation, Stjernswärd and I planned to spend 2 years field-testing the effectiveness of the proposed WHO method with multinational trials conducted in the five countries that had been involved in the original study and under the aegis of the WHO collaborating centers in Milan and Boston. A major meeting would then be held in Geneva, after which a comprehensive report with full recommendations on the management of cancer pain would be published by WHO. In fact, at the time of the Geneva meeting, useful progress had been made in only one of the studies we had hoped to be completed. The results were reported by Fumikazu Takeda of the Saitama Cancer Center in Japan, where 87% of the 156 patients treated by the "ladder" method reported complete freedom from pain. In the years since then, a large number of reports have confirmed the undoubted value of the method.

Another element of our planning at this stage was consideration of the logistical problems that would be involved in the dissemination of our cancer pain relief program. Thus we had to promote the supply of drugs to and within the less developed parts of the world, the easing of legal restrictions on opioid importation and use, and the need for education of doctors, medical students, and nurses in the appropriate use of strong narcotics. At that time (1984), the use of oral opiates was not widely permitted even in many Western countries due to restrictive governmental regulations, many of them enacted as a result of the work of WHO's own Expert Committee on Drugs Liable to Produce Addiction. In the years that followed, we worked hard on contacting and persuading national ministries of health that ours was a worthwhile project and on overcoming the problems of narcotic drug control. This important endeavor has been continued since my retirement by David Joranson of the WHO Collaborating Center at the University of Wisconsin.

The meeting at WHO headquarters in Geneva on December 11–14, 1984, was key to promoting the program. In addition to many of the participants of the Milan meeting, the delegates included representatives of ministries of health and cancer research units in China, Finland, France, West Germany, Nigeria, Sri Lanka, the Netherlands, the United Kingdom, and the Soviet Union, as well as observers from the International Federation of Pharmaceutical Manufacturers Associations, the IASP, the World Federation of Cancer Care, and the International Union Against Cancer.

The results of the conference's deliberations were written up as a small handbook entitled *Cancer Pain Relief* by Twycross and Stjernswärd and published by WHO in 1986. This booklet was translated into 15 languages and distributed worldwide within 2 years. *Cancer Pain Relief* explains the principles of the method advocated and points out that analgesic drugs are effective in most patients when used correctly—the right drug in the right dose at the right time intervals—and that they can be used without risk of abuse or psychological dependence in most patients. The booklet explains different pain syndromes and makes it clear that some cancer pains are best treated by a combination of drug and nondrug methods.

The three primary analgesics recommended are aspirin (alternatively acetaminophen), codeine (alternatively dextropropoxyphene), and morphine (alternatively methadone, meperidine, or buprenorphine). The alternative routes of administration that may be necessary are detailed. The booklet also describes the adjuvant drugs that should be used when necessary to deal with specific types of pain and to help with other discomforts, namely anticonvulsants, neurolytics, anxiolytics, antidepressants, and corticosteroids. In 1987, Ventafridda and I published a book on cancer pain (Swerdlow and Ventafridda 1987) that covers in greater detail the appropriate management of cancer pain both by drug and nondrug measures.

As the years have gone by, the cancer unit has continued to spread knowledge of the pain relief method, in cooperation particularly with the IASP, and has kept a keen watch on the vast number of publications reporting clinical trials of the ladder technique. It has also continued to encourage all nations to implement effective cancer pain relief measures. The success of these efforts is reflected by the large number of health ministries and national organizations of health professionals that have agreed to adopt the WHO cancer pain relief program. WHO is also giving increasing attention to the subject of palliative care.

REFERENCES

Bonica JJ. Introductory statement to the symposium on cancer pain: importance of the problem. In: Bonica JJ, Ventafridda V, Fink BR, Jones LE, Loeser JD (Eds). *Proceedings of the First International Symposium on Pain in Advanced Cancer,* Advances in Pain Research and Therapy, Vol. 2. New York: Raven Press, 1979, pp 1–2.

Swerdlow M (Comp). Responses to WHO physician questionnaires. *Mark Swerdlow Papers,* John C. Licbeskind History of Pain Collection, Louise M. Darling Biomedical Library, University of California, Los Angeles, 1981.

Swerdlow M, Stjernswärd J. Cancer pain relief: an urgent problem. *World Health Forum* 1982; 3:329.

Swerdlow M, Ventafridda V. *Cancer Pain.* Boston: MTP Press, 1987.

World Health Organization. *Cancer Pain Relief.* Geneva: World Health Organization, 1986.

Correspondence to: Marcia L. Meldrum, PhD, Department of History, Bunche 6265, Box 951473, University of California, Los Angeles, Los Angeles, CA 90095-1473, USA. Email: meldrum@history.ucla.edu.

Opioids and Pain Relief: A Historical Perspective,
Progress in Pain Research and Management, Vol.
25, edited by Marcia L. Meldrum, IASP Press,
Seattle, © 2003.

12

The State Cancer Pain Initiative Movement in the United States: Successes and Challenges

June L. Dahl

*Department of Pharmacology, University of Wisconsin
Medical School, Madison, Wisconsin, USA*

This chapter discusses the formation and evolution of state cancer pain initiatives. These organizations, which have formed in the majority of states in the United States, are dedicated to improving the management of cancer pain. I will discuss their origins, the successes they have achieved, and the special challenges they face, and provide some perspectives on the role that these initiatives can and should play in current pain management improvement efforts in the United States. This discussion reflects my personal journey of almost 20 years, because my involvement with pain management improvement efforts is intimately linked to the cancer pain initiative movement. It has been exciting to watch pain management become a priority in this country and to witness the dramatic changes that have occurred since the first state cancer pain initiative was formed in Wisconsin in 1986 (Dahl et al. 1988). At the same time, it is sobering to recognize that despite the dedication of so many individuals working within and outside this program, much of the pain of cancer still is not effectively managed. Studies continue to document that more than half of all patients with advanced cancer endure moderate to severe pain (Weiss et al. 2001).

WHAT ARE STATE CANCER PAIN INITIATIVES?

State cancer pain initiatives are volunteer interdisciplinary efforts involving physicians, nurses, pharmacists, social workers, psychologists, educators, clergy, drug regulators, and representatives of state government agencies who are dedicated to improving the management of cancer pain. Such inclusiveness is an important characteristic of these organizations and reflects the diversity of skills and knowledge needed to address the multidimensional aspects of pain management. State-based efforts make sense because the education, regulation, and licensing of health care professionals occur at the state level, as do the regulation and licensing of certain health care facilities. For example, state agencies survey long-term care facilities, home health agencies, and some community hospitals to determine whether they meet standards that render them eligible to receive federal funds to support care of the elderly and disabled. Because the United States is a large, demographically and geographically diverse nation, state-based organizations can take advantage of the particular strengths and confront the unique challenges inherent within each region.

ORIGINS OF THE INITIATIVE MOVEMENT

The Wisconsin Cancer Pain Initiative (WCPI) has a unique history. Created by the state's drug regulatory authority, the Wisconsin Controlled Substances Board (WCSB), it emerged as a response to a bill that was introduced into the U.S. Congress in 1984 to enact the Compassionate Pain Relief Act, which would allow medical use of heroin (diamorphine) to treat pain in terminally ill cancer patients. Members of Congress who had seen their loved ones die in agony from cancer, and who knew that heroin was used in British hospices, believed erroneously that the drug was a "magic bullet" that would prevent cancer patients from having to die in pain.

In 1984, I was serving as chair of the WCSB. That summer, our family took a vacation trip from Madison to Washington, DC. The very first day we were there, the *Washington Post* published an editorial in support of the Compassionate Pain Relief Act, which aroused my concern. Although I was unable to gain access to the newspaper's editorial offices, I did visit the offices of Wisconsin's congressional delegation. I tried to explain that heroin's availability would not resolve the problem of pain in patients receiving curative treatment, and that research had shown that administration of heroin was an expensive and controversial way to deliver morphine (Dahl and Joranson 1993). My arguments fell on deaf ears. A typical response from a staff member was: "The Congressman's aunt died in agony from cancer; he doesn't want anyone else to suffer. He is convinced that the answer is heroin, because after all, look at the success that the British hospices are having with heroin in Brompton's cocktail." The message was clear: "Don't bother us with the facts, our minds are made up." Indeed, I have received similar responses when discussing other issues related to pain management. Emotions about this difficult problem can easily sweep away attempts to craft responses based on evidence.

I returned to Wisconsin frustrated, and convinced of the need for a more effective response to the cancer pain problem. There was no question that pain was poorly treated. As chair of the WCSB, I was fortunate to have as a colleague and board member David Joranson, who has worked tirelessly since the late 1980s to improve the availability of opioids in many countries of the world. We decided to oppose the "heroin bill" and conveyed that position to members of Congress. The bill did not pass. However, the board recognized that its own actions might have contributed to the cancer pain problem: it had developed a vigorous program to prevent the diversion and abuse of prescription controlled substances, particularly opioids, and had told Wisconsin physicians that they should exercise great caution when prescribing those drugs. If they did not, they were likely to face a reprimand by the state's regulatory authorities. The WCSB determined that if it were part of the problem, it should become part of the solution, and decided to couple its opposition to the "heroin bill" with a positive response: to develop a comprehensive program to improve management of cancer pain in the state. Initially we called ourselves the Wisconsin Initiative for Improving Cancer Pain Management.

In a preliminary proposal we outlined critical elements of a plan for action:

1) The focus should be on pain at all stages of the disease and not be limited to the terminally ill. (This focus is even more important today because with advances in treatment, cancer has become a chronic disease, and patients are living longer and longer with pain. Furthermore, persons may be cured of their disease, but remain in pain because of the effects of treatments.)

2) Undertreatment is not due to a lack of effective therapies; the problem is that they were not being used appropriately. (Unfortunately, this is still an issue. Despite significant advances in the science and medicine of pain since the mid-1980s, application of that new knowledge lags behind.)

3) Educational programs have not changed clinical practice. Knowledge is critical, but knowledge alone does not change behaviors.

4) Any program to improve pain management must address the need to change the attitudes and behaviors of health care professionals.

5) A program developed in Wisconsin should be sufficiently comprehensive to be useful to persons in other states.

Between 1984 and 1986, we began to lay the foundation by engaging individual clinicians, medical and nursing schools, professional societies, and various state agencies, and by forming a steering committee. Recognizing that the nursing organizations had never collaborated, we brought them together. We invited pharmacists to a separate dialogue because they presented some unique challenges to improving opioid availability and appropriate use.

After 2 years of preparation, the board hosted a strategic planning session in December 1986. A stellar group of invited guests spoke to the importance of our actions: Jan Stjernswärd, Chief of the Cancer Unit of the World Health Organization (WHO); Kathleen Foley, Chief of the Pain Service at Memorial Sloan Kettering Cancer Center in New York; John C. Duffy, Assistant Surgeon General of the United States; a spokesperson from the National Institute on Drug Abuse; and pain management advocates from India and Mexico (Dahl et al. 1988).

Under Stjernswärd's leadership, WHO had made pain relief a key priority of its cancer program; its 1986 publication, *Cancer Pain Relief*, documented the worldwide problem and introduced the concept of the "analgesic ladder" (World Health Organization 1986). At that December meeting and much to our delight, Stjernswärd named the WCPI a demonstration project of WHO. We have carried that designation with pride as we have watched the growth of efforts to improve pain management throughout the world.

Health professionals, state officials, and laypersons in other states soon showed interest in developing cancer pain initiatives. The Second World Congress on Cancer Pain, held in Rye, New York, in the summer of 1988, provided an opportunity for dialogue. I gave a brief description of the WCPI during a session on WHO cancer pain relief efforts, and more importantly, joined my colleagues in discussing the WCPI during a workshop. Clinicians who attended began to plan pain initiatives in their home areas. In 1989, the WCPI hosted a national meeting of persons interested in forming pain initiatives; six delegates took the message home and organized initiatives in their own states shortly thereafter. In 1992, the Robert Wood Johnson Foundation provided funding to create the Resource Center for State Pain Initiatives in Madison, which stimulated rapid growth of pain initiatives during the 1990s. This foundation, the largest philanthropic organization in the United States dedicated to making improvements in health care, has provided significant additional funding to support pain initiative projects. Its generosity has made possible several critical projects and has helped to make end-of-life care a priority in the United States (Gibson 1998).

In 1996, members of this growing movement formed a national organization, the American Alliance of Cancer Pain Initiatives (AACPI), to provide a communications network, to share resources, to give the movement a national identity, and to permit initiatives to speak with a common voice (Dahl 1996). The AACPI sponsors an annual national meeting that is the only forum to focus specifically on the organizational, ethical, cultural, educational, and policy challenges surrounding the treatment of cancer pain.

Collaboration has always been key to pain initiative activities. In 2001, the AACPI established a formal collaborative relationship with the American Cancer Society, which has broadened its goals beyond prevention and curative therapy to include quality of life, with pain management as a key component (American Cancer Society 2001). The unique strengths of the two organizations provide a perfect complement to each other. The state initiatives have expertise about pain control, access to health care providers, and a passion for reducing the burden of pain. The American Cancer Society has a rich history of service and excellent name recognition and brings fund-raising proficiency, advocacy skills, and expertise in organizing meetings. We have also collaborated with cancer centers, hospice organizations, and professional schools.

WHAT IS THE FOCUS OF STATEWIDE PAIN MANAGEMENT IMPROVEMENT EFFORTS?

Initiatives focus their efforts on overcoming the barriers to effective pain management. Survey research has documented problems related to health care professionals; patients, families, and the public at large; the health care system; the drug regulatory system; and the reimbursement system (Pargeon and Hailey 1999). Pioneering studies by Charles Cleeland provided the basis for the WCPI action plan. For example, his research revealed that more than half of the patients with advanced cancer who were receiving treatment at the University of Wisconsin's Comprehensive Cancer Center had moderate to severe pain (Daut and Cleeland 1982). He also demonstrated how lack of knowledge and inappropriate attitudes of health care professionals contribute to the undertreatment of pain (Cleeland 1987). Health care professionals had (and still have) excessive concerns about opioid side effects, especially about the potential for addiction. I would never want to diminish the importance of the nation's drug abuse problem, but there is no evidence that addiction is a problem in those with chronic cancer pain who require long-term opioid therapy. However, apprehension still surrounds even the routine use of opioids, a fear that Morgan (1989) has called *opiophobia.* The recent media frenzy about the diversion and abuse of controlled-release oxycodone (OxyContin) has exacerbated fears about addiction and the abuse of opioid analgesics (Ziegler and Lovrich 2002; Acker, this volume).

Professional education. Initiatives have held numerous conferences and workshops to improve knowledge and change attitudes of health care professionals. During the 1990s, the WCPI sponsored Cancer Pain Role Model Programs in 26 states that brought together teams of physicians and nurses to teach them the basics of pain management and to help them develop plans for changing pain practices in their care settings (Weissman and Dahl 1995). The New Jersey Pain Initiative sponsored Best Practices Programs that reached 1,500 health care professionals during the 13 months ending in December 2000. Other initiatives host annual or semiannual meetings for clinicians in all the disciplines involved in the care of patients in pain (Dahl et al. 2002).

Patient education. Sandra Ward of the University of Wisconsin School of Nursing has identified important patient-related barriers to effective cancer pain control (Ward et al. 1993). She showed that patients feel that pain is inevitable with cancer. They may believe that talking about their pain will distract their doctors from curing their disease, and that they should save their medicine until the pain "really gets bad." Because of their desire to be "good" patients, they are reluctant to "complain" (i.e., to report their pain), and they are worried about getting addicted if they are treated with "strong" pain medicine. Critical to Ward's research is her finding that the more strongly patients adhered to these beliefs, the less likely they were to receive adequate pain management.

The initiatives' message to patients and families is available in print and audio formats and also via the Internet (www.wisc.edu/wcpi). This information assures patients that cancer pain can be controlled, that they have the right to effective control of their pain, that addiction is not an issue when cancer patients take opioids for pain control, and that good pain control means better cancer control. Initiatives have also worked to dispel the myth that aggressive pain control shortens life (Wall 1997).

Public education. Efforts to improve the knowledge of the public have also been important. In 1998, Cancer Pain Relief Utah engaged in a successful public relations campaign. In collaboration with the Community State Partnerships to Improve End-of-Life Care and the Utah Broadcasters Association, the organization broadcast key messages on 35 stations. In 2001, a video feed that highlighted the importance of good pain control and new pain standards for the nation's health care facilities reached 11 million viewers. AACPI plans to expand its public education efforts through collaboration with the American Pain Foundation (www.painfoundation.org), an organization founded in 1997 to serve persons with pain and improve their quality of life by raising public awareness, providing practical information, promoting research, and advocating the removal of barriers and increased access to effective pain management.

The health care system. Perhaps the most formidable barriers are presented by the health care system itself. Pain has had low priority in medical practice. There has been little accountability for poor pain management;

clinicians have not assessed pain and have lacked access to practical treatment protocols. Care is often fragmented and uncoordinated as patients move from one health care setting to another. Initiatives have addressed this problem through "institutional change" programs, with the goal of changing the culture of the health care facilities that take care of persons with pain. WCPI published a manual, *Building an Institutional Commitment to Pain Management* (Gordon et al. 2000), based on principles articulated by the American Pain Society Quality of Care Committee (1995) and other groups. The manual was designed to help health care facilities make the structural changes essential to ensure that pain management becomes an integral part of patient care.

The critical next step was to engage the Joint Commission on Accreditation of Healthcare Organizations (JCAHO), the major accrediting body in the United States. JCAHO accredits 80% of the nation's hospitals, accounting for 96% of inpatient admissions. The commission also accredits behavioral health facilities, long-term care facilities, and home health agencies, so it has great potential to influence the quality of pain management in the United States. Health care facilities use their JCAHO accreditation to obtain "deemed status" and thus qualify for federal Medicaid and Medicare funding. The JCAHO pain standards, requiring pain assessment of every patient, were released in the summer of 1999, and became a formal part of the survey and accreditation process in January 2001 (Joint Commission on Accreditation of Healthcare Organizations 2000).

The AACPI has assisted health care facilities in many states to meet JCAHO requirements through programs aimed at making pain management an institutional priority. It has sponsored Practice Change Programs in eight states; these programs engage long-term care facilities, home health agencies, and community hospitals in a given geographic area of a state in a year-long program aimed at changing pain management practices in the various care settings (Stevenson et al. 2002).

Regulatory barriers. Controlled substances regulations have been identified as important barriers to effective pain control (Joranson and Gilson 1998). Although federal laws do not impede the appropriate use of opioids for pain control, many states have promulgated regulations that can have a chilling effect on the prescribing and dispensing of controlled substances. Therefore, state pain initiatives have worked to remove regulatory barriers in the states and have promoted adoption of the model guidelines developed by the Federation of State Medical Boards (1998) for the use of opioids. The initiatives work closely with the Pain and Policy Studies Group at the University of Wisconsin (www.medsch.wisc.edu/painpolicy), directed by Joranson, and use the results of its comprehensive analysis of state policies to craft strategies for improving the "regulatory climate" in individual states (Pain and Policy Studies Group 2000).

The AACPI participated in the development of a position statement from the Drug Enforcement Administration (DEA), the agency that administers the Federal Controlled Substances Act, and 44 health organizations. The position statement emphasizes the importance of balancing the need for the use of opioids for good pain control with the need to prevent their diversion and abuse (Dahl 2002).

Reimbursement barriers. Reimbursement policies present another potential set of barriers. There is no system of universal health care in the United States; 40 million persons in the United States have no health insurance, insurance premiums are increasingly expensive, and various insurance plans limit coverage in uniquely restrictive ways. They may pay for a $10,000 pump for delivery of spinal opioids, but not cover an in-home nurse's visit to teach a patient how to take medications orally. They may not pay for complementary therapies such as massage and acupuncture. Many of the newer drugs and drug formulations are very expensive and are not covered by private insurance plans, nor by federally funded Medicare programs. State initiatives, often working in collaboration with the American Cancer Society, have challenged some of the inequities. The Virginia Cancer Pain Initiative was successful in advocating legislation to improve terminally ill patients' access to health care services. Virginia law now requires all health maintenance organizations to pay for pain medications, to cover access to hospice services, and to allow patients access to pain specialists and oncologists without a referral (Dahl et al. 2002).

CURRENT STATUS OF THE PAIN INITIATIVE MOVEMENT

Initiatives have now formed in 44 states. Their size and strengths vary greatly. In some states the initiative is best described as a collection of dedicated individuals; in other states such as California, it is a well-established force for change. Initiatives in 15 states have decided to address all types of pain, both acute and chronic, and have dropped the word "cancer" from their name. The WCPI, for example, is now called the Wisconsin Pain Initiative.

We were extremely naive in 1986 in believing that we could solve the cancer pain problem in about 5 years. Perhaps this attitude was fortunate, because otherwise we might never have started on what has turned out to be an amazing journey. As we overcome one set of barriers, others seem to arise, and new obstacles continue to challenge us. We are still involved in educating health care professionals, but we have expanded our efforts to promote institutional change because we recognized that education alone does not change practice (Max 1990). We continue to raise public and patient awareness of the cancer pain problem and to help patients understand that effective pain control is good for them and that pain does not build character or make anyone a better person. We want everyone to understand that unrelieved pain has no redeeming virtues. We continue to work to remove regulatory and legislative barriers and to disseminate accurate pain management information. We are challenged because perceptions so often hold sway over reality. The Wisconsin Pain Initiative has embarked on a new venture to determine what barriers may prevent appropriate payment for pain treatment in the state. We hear anecdotal reports that payment systems often discourage and in some instances even prevent access to pain relief. But we must document that this is true if we are to present our case successfully to policy makers.

We are committed to increasing the cultural diversity of the state initiatives. The AACPI network now includes a Native American cancer pain initiative known as the Unbroken Circle Initiative. Native Americans with cancer often do not seek health care until their disease is advanced; at the very least, we must provide symptom control to such patients. Many cultural barriers make it particularly challenging to provide effective pain control for native peoples (Elliott et al. 1999). The AACPI now has a seat on the Board of Directors of the Intercultural Cancer Council (www.iccnetwork.org), an organization that promotes policies, programs, partnerships, and research to eliminate the unequal burden of cancer among racial and ethnic minorities, and on other medically underserved populations in the United States and its territories.

WHAT OF THE FUTURE?

When the WCPI was formed in 1986, no national efforts were dedicated to bringing improvements in the management of cancer pain. Although the American hospice movement had begun in Connecticut in 1972, its philosophy did not quickly capture the interest of an American public and a medical profession that seemed bent on defying and denying death. Finally, in the early 1990s, we saw increasing recognition of the importance of effective pain control with position statements from the Oncology Nursing Society (Spross et al. 1990) and the American Society of Clinical Oncology (American Society of Clinical Oncology Ad Hoc Committee on Cancer Pain 1992). The past decade also witnessed the development of the American Academy of Pain Medicine for physicians and the American Society of Pain Management

Nurses. Numerous evidence-based pain guidelines have been published, including one specifically dealing with cancer pain (Agency for Health Care Policy and Research 1994). The JCAHO pain standards mean that no accredited facility can ignore pain. In the summer of 2002, the National Institutes of Health sponsored a State-of-the-Science Conference on Symptom Management in Cancer: Pain, Depression and Fatigue, which urged that greater resources be dedicated to providing relief of the symptoms of the disease (National Institutes of Health 2002). Other efforts have focused on acute pain and persistent pain unrelated to cancer (e.g., American Geriatrics Society Panel on Persistent Pain in Older Persons 2002). Advances in the science and medicine of pain have been impressive, with novel drugs, new drug delivery systems, technologically sophisticated approaches to treatment, and recognition of the critical importance of nonpharmacological methods of pain control.

Do these accomplishments make the pain initiative movement obsolete? Many organizations are finally giving pain the attention it has so long deserved. Should we abdicate our role, given our limited resources? Such questions force us to reflect on our strengths, our challenges, and the unique niche that we occupy because we have no crystal ball to help us predict the future. We can draw upon our strengths: (1) a network of committed individuals in the states, persons with expertise and passion; (2) the demonstrated ability to collaborate and network with others who share the common goal of assuring pain relief for all persons with cancer; and (3) our interdisciplinary nature, which allows us to bring a great breadth and depth of expertise and skills to our work.

We acknowledge the challenges of limited human and material resources, as well as the volunteer nature of many state pain initiatives, which often lack paid staff and rely upon the energies of overworked health care professionals. One solution may be tap into the pool of American Cancer Society volunteers who serve that organization so well. Another problem is the enormous size of the nation. In particular, the sparse populations of central and mountain states mean that access to appropriate care can be limited by distance rather than by financial resources.

Whatever our challenges, no other organizations are dedicated to working at the state level. Each state presents unique challenges that cannot be properly addressed by national mandates. Finally, I believe that the current crisis in health care delivery increases the need for independent knowledgeable and forceful advocacy groups to promote adequate pain relief for all persons.

ACKNOWLEDGMENTS

This paper is dedicated to the memory of Dr. John Liebeskind, whose research advanced our knowledge of basic pain mechanisms, whose foresight led to the establishment of the UCLA History of Pain Project, and whose kind and generous spirit touched us all. I gratefully acknowledge the support the Robert Wood Johnson Foundation has provided to the state pain initiative movement.

REFERENCES

Agency for Health Care Policy and Research. *Management of Cancer Pain: Adults.* Clinical Practice Guideline No. 9, AHCPR Publication No. 94-0593. Rockville, MD: U.S. Public Health Service, Agency for Health Care Policy and Research, 1994.

American Cancer Society. *Implementing Pain Management Initiatives: A Resource Book for Divisions.* Atlanta, GA: American Cancer Society, 2001.

American Geriatrics Society Panel on Persistent Pain in Older Persons. The management of persistent pain in older persons. *J Am Geriatr Soc* 2002; 50:S205–224.

American Pain Society Quality of Care Committee. Quality improvement guidelines for the treatment of acute pain and cancer pain. *JAMA* 1995; 274:1874–1880.

American Society of Clinical Oncology Ad Hoc Committee on Cancer Pain. Cancer pain assessment and treatment curriculum guidelines. *J Clin Oncol* 1992; 10:1976–1982.

Cleeland CS. Barriers to the management of cancer pain. *Oncology* 1987; Suppl:19–26.

Dahl JL. State initiatives form a national organization: the American Alliance of Cancer Pain Initiatives. *APS Bull* 1996; 6:3.

Dahl JL. Working with regulators to improve the standard of care in pain management: the U.S. experience. *J Pain Symptom Manage* 2002; 24:136–147.

Dahl JL, Joranson DE. Heroin and cancer pain initiatives. *Am J Hosp Pharm* 1993; 50:2060–2061.

Dahl JL, Joranson DE, Engber D, Dosch J. The cancer pain problem: Wisconsin's response. *J Pain Symptom Manage* 1988; 3:S1–S20.

Dahl JL, Bennett ME, Bromley MD, Joranson DE. Success of the state pain initiatives: moving pain management forward. *Cancer Pract* 2002; 10:S9–S13.

Daut RI, Cleeland CS. The prevalence and severity of pain in cancer. *Cancer* 1982; 50:1913–1918.

Elliott BA, Johnson KM, Elliott TE, Day JJ. Enhancing cancer pain control among American Indians (ECPCAI): a study of the Ojibwe of Minnesota. *J Cancer Educ* 1999; 14:28–33.

Federation of State Medical Boards of the United States. *Model Guidelines for the Use of Controlled Substances for the Treatment of Pain.* Euless, TX: Federation of State Medical Boards of the United States, 1998.

Gibson R. The Robert Wood Johnson Foundation grant-making strategies to improve end-of-life care. *J Palliat Med* 1998; 1:415–417.

Gordon DB, Dahl JL, Stevenson KK. *Building an Institutional Commitment to Pain Management: the Wisconsin Resource Manual.* Madison, WI: University of Wisconsin Madison Board of Regents, 2000.

Joranson DE, Gilson AM. Regulatory barriers to pain management. *Semin Oncol Nurs* 1998; 14:158–163.

Joint Commission on Accreditation for Healthcare Organizations. *Comprehensive Accreditation Manual for Hospitals.* Oakbrook Terrace, IL: Joint Commission on Accreditation for Healthcare Organizations, 2000.

Max M. Improving outcomes of analgesic treatment: Is education enough? *Ann Intern Med* 1990; 113:885–889.

Morgan JP. American opiophobia: customary underutilization of opioid analgesics. In: Hill CS Jr, Fields WS (Eds). *Drug Treatment of Cancer Pain in a Drug-Oriented Society,* Advances in Pain Research and Therapy, Vol. 11. New York: Raven Press, 1989, pp 181–189.

National Institutes of Health. Available via the Internet: consensus.nih.gov. Accessed December 2002.

Pain and Policy Studies Group. *Achieving Balance in Federal and State Pain Policy: A Guide to Evaluation.* Madison, WI: University of Wisconsin-Madison, 2000.

Pargeon KL, Hailey BJ. Barriers to effective cancer pain management: a review of the literature. *J Pain Symptom Manage* 1999; 18:358–368.

Spross JA, McGuire DB, Schmitt RM. Oncology Nursing Society position paper on cancer pain. *Oncol Nurs Forum* 1990; 17:595–614, 751–760, 943–955.

Stevenson KM, Berry PH, Griffie J, Muchka SL, Dahl JL. Using practice change programs to improve pain management. *Abstracts: 10th World Congress on Pain.* Seattle: IASP Press, 2002, pp 226–227.

Wall PD. The generation of another myth on the use of narcotics. *Pain* 1997; 73:121–122.

Ward SE, Goldberg N, Miller-McCauley V, et al. Patient related barriers to management of cancer pain. *Pain* 1993; 52:319–324.

Weiss SC, Emanuel LL, Fairclough DL, Emanuel EJ. Understanding the experience of pain in terminally ill patients. *Lancet* 2001; 357:1311–1315.

Weissman DE, Dahl JL. Update on the cancer pain role model education program. *J Pain Symptom Manage* 1995; 10:292–297.

World Health Organization. *Cancer Pain Relief.* Geneva: World Health Organization, 1986.

Ziegler SJ, Lovrich NP. OxyContin and the need for perspective. *Pain and the Law* 2002. Available via the Internet: www.painandthelaw.org/mayday/Ziegler_lovrich_010702.php.

Correspondence to: June L. Dahl, PhD, University of Wisconsin Medical School, 4735 Medical Sciences Center, 1300 University Avenue, Madison, WI 53706, USA. Email: jldahl@facstaff.wisc.edu.

Opioids and Pain Relief: A Historical Perspective,
Progress in Pain Research and Management, Vol.
25, edited by Marcia L. Meldrum, IASP Press,
Seattle, © 2003.

13

Opioids, Cancer Pain, Quality of Life, and Quality of Death: Patient Narratives and a Clinician's Comments

Nessa Coyle

Department of Neurology, Pain and Palliative Care Service,
Memorial-Sloan-Kettering Cancer Center, New York, New York, USA

Pain continues to be undertreated despite an ever-growing list of options and methods for its relief and the availability of effective pharmacological and nonpharmacological approaches. Although pain has become recognized in the last several years as an avoidable public health problem (Institute of Medicine 1997; Joint Commission on Accreditation of Healthcare Organizations 2000), chronic unrelieved pain continues to exhaust many patients, their families, and professional caregivers, leaving them demoralized and disheartened. Unrelieved severe pain has a devastating effect, not only on patients but also on those close to them. It can lead patients to desire death and family and caregivers to feel that death would indeed be a blessing. The increased availability of opioid drugs and other techniques should have made episodes of unrelieved pain largely a thing of the past; however, this is not the experience of many patients. The reasons are varied and complex.

Numerous surveys over the past several decades have identified barriers that interfere with adequate pain management (Levin et al. 1985; Grossman et al. 1991; Gonzales and Coyle 1992; Von Roenn et al. 1993; Cleeland et al. 1994; Jacox et al. 1994; Cherny and Catane 1995; Pargeon and Hailey 1999). These barriers have been broadly characterized as clinician related, health care system related, and patient and family related. Clinician-related barriers include inadequate knowledge of pain management, poor assessment of pain, concerns about regulation of controlled substances, fear of patient addiction, worries about side effects of analgesics, and concerns about patients becoming tolerant to analgesics. Surveys have demonstrated the failure of clinicians to evaluate or appreciate the severity of the pain problem (Grossman et al. 1991; Von Roenn et al. 1993; Wallace et al. 1995). Indeed, inaccurate assessment of pain severity may be a major predictor of inadequate relief.

Barriers related to the health care system include lack of visibility of pain; lack of a common language to describe pain; lack of commitment to pain management as a priority; restrictive regulation of controlled substances; economic factors; problems of availability of treatment or access to it, especially in minority communities; and failure to use validated measurement tools in clinical practice (Joranson et al. 1992; Bookbinder et al. 1995; Foley 1998; Anderson et al. 2000, 2002; Gunnarsdottir et al. 2002). Further complications are patient- and family-related barriers, including reluctance to report pain, unwillingness to follow treatment recommendations, fears of tolerance and addiction, concerns about opioid-related side effects, fears about disease progression, belief that pain is an inevitable part of cancer and must be accepted, and cost of the analgesics.

Recognition of family-related barriers in the use of opioids is extraordinarily important because most chronic pain is both experienced and managed in the home (Coyle 2001). Families of the chronically ill and dying play a key role in deciding whether the patient will take prescribed opioid drugs. An early small descriptive study (describing 10 cases) that investigated the experience of managing pain at home from the perspective of the patient, the primary family caregiver, and the home care nurse encapsulates many of the important areas that affect pain management in the home (Taylor et al. 1993). The main areas of decision making and conflict centered around the use of opioid medications. Patients were preoccupied with decisions about the type of medication and the optimal dose. Adverse side effects and negative conceptual images of opioids contributed to mental conflicts in patients who wondered whether they were doing the "right thing" in taking the pain medication. Similarly, the conflicts that arose most frequently for family caregivers also related to opioid drugs and decisions about which pill to give and when to give it. Compounding these difficulties were concerns about overdosing, adverse side effects, and addiction. In a study by Ward et al. (1996) that evaluated these patient- and family-related barriers, a higher level of concern was correlated with the undermedication of pain.

In the majority of all barriers related to undertreatment of pain, the underlying theme is concern about the use of opioid drugs. And yet these drugs are the mainstay of cancer pain treatment.

A CLINICIAN'S EXPERIENCE WITH OPIOIDS
OVER THREE DECADES

I have worked as a pain and palliative care clinician over the past three decades. Care of advanced cancer patients has been the focus of my practice, and encounters with patients suffering from both chronic and acute pain are a daily challenge. The availability of a range of opioid drugs, different preparations and diverse routes of administration, and information about equianalgesic dose ratios when switching from a particular drug or route of administration to another have made a huge difference in my ability to control pain associated with cancer and its treatment. For some cancer patients, however, the management of opioid-related side effects in the setting of rapidly advancing disease remains extremely difficult.

The principles of the pharmacological management of pain have remained simple and unchanged over the years: believe the patient's statement of pain; know the pharmacology of the drug and time action curve; select a drug and route of administration based on pain severity and the patient's analgesic history and medical state; administer the drug on a regular basis for chronic pain, providing "rescue" medication for breakthrough pain; assess the effectiveness of pain relief and presence of adverse side effects; titrate the opioid drug to achieve good pain relief with minimal adverse side effects, rotating opioids if indicated; and aggressively treat adverse side effects if they occur. Patients and families, however, continue to worry about psychological dependence, the inability to control future pain, and cognitive or gastrointestinal side effects when opioid drugs are introduced or escalated to manage pain. Perhaps the presence or possibility of cognitive side effects, of "loss of self," gives rise to the deepest concern.

Societal concern about opioid drugs as a class is reflected in their limited availability in some community pharmacies (Kanner and Portenoy 1986; Morrison et al. 2000; Resnik 2001). In the United States, for example, special prescriptions are required in many states for ordering opioid drugs, and renewals are not permitted without a new prescription. Families are warned to keep these drugs in a safe place and out of reach of children. When a patient requires higher doses of an opioid than is customary in the community health care network, a pharmacist or other concerned professional may warn the patient and family member of the dangers and question the appropriateness of such a dose. All of these factors reinforce a general sense of unease in all but the most seasoned pain and palliative care practitioner, an unease readily imparted to the patient and family.

The involvement of patient and family and their agreement that the proposed pain management plan will serve the patient's best interest underscore the success of any treatment approach. When deciding which approach is best, families carefully weigh the goals of the patient's care and the possible side effects of treatment that might impinge on these goals. When the clinical situation or goals of care change, the patient and family may readily accept an approach that once was unacceptable.

THE PATIENT'S EXPERIENCE OF CANCER-RELATED PAIN AND USE OF OPIOIDS

The prevalence of pain in the individual with cancer varies by diagnosis and other factors. Approximately one-third of patients undergoing cancer therapy and two-thirds of those with advanced disease experience pain (Daut and Cleeland 1982; Ng and von Gunten 1998). Almost three-quarters of patients with advanced cancer admitted to the hospital are in pain at the time of admission (Brescia et al. 1992). Efforts have been made to define the interface between pain and suffering (Fishman 1991; Foley 1991; Cherny and Coyle 1994; Cherny and Portenoy 1994). In clinical situations the question "What does this pain mean to you" or the use of the word "morphine" to name the tool to control their pain may release a verbal flood of suffering and fear from both patient and family.

This chapter analyzes the narratives of seven individuals living with advanced cancer who described how both pain and the use of opioid drugs affected their quality of life, and uses their words to illustrate how they viewed the mainstay of cancer pain treatment—opioid drugs—as both a blessing and a burden. These narratives come from a study that was part of a phenomenological inquiry on the experience of living with advanced cancer and how that experience affects attitudes toward life and death (N. Coyle, unpublished manuscript). One of the criteria for acceptance into the study was that patients had expressed at least once a desire for hastened death. The goal of the study was to identify the grounds for such an expression. The experiences presented are those of the patients, not of their family or caregivers, who may have experienced the same situation differently.

SEVEN CANCER PATIENTS TELL THEIR STORY

Vinnie, Connie, Myra, Archie, Harry, Diana, and Larry were living with advanced cancer. They had received most of their medical care at an urban cancer research center. Their backgrounds were diverse, but what they all had in common was a desire for continued life, despite having at least once expressed a desire for death. Episodes of severe physical pain were part of their cancer experience. Pain dominated some conversations with compelling intensity and emotionality. The issues surrounding their pain experience were varied and complex.

Vinnie and Myra, for example, were concerned about the consequences of acknowledging uncontrolled pain because of the possibility that pain would then become the focus of their care, which they feared might reduce their eligibility for possible life-prolonging chemotherapy regimens. Others spoke of the impact of severe pain on their will to live, stating that the fear of pain was sometimes greater than the fear of death itself. For some, their own encounter with pain brought back memories of uncontrolled pain in a loved one. Pain was a reminder of the progression of disease and the imminence of death, and sometimes led to expressions of anger toward and confusion about God, and soul-searching about why such pain was allowed to happen.

Connie and Archie expressed great concern that the side effects of opioid therapy would make them sleepy or dull their minds. All seven patients, while still striving to live, were also making great efforts to ensure good pain relief when dying; they chose a site of care that offered the greatest possibilities to ensure a comfortable death and where caregivers would "dial up the morphine" to whatever level necessary to ensure pain relief. They saw opioid use as a guarantor of a peaceful death, and some of them perceived opioids as a welcome means of hastening death.

These narratives, showing that patients view the use of opioid drugs as both a blessing and a burden, reflect typical encounters in daily clinical practice. The "blessing" in these narratives reflects freedom from pain, while poorly controlled adverse side effects such as sleepiness or mental clouding constitute the "burden." Without exception, however, as death drew near, patients saw the availability of potent opioid drugs as a blessing. The themes outlined below illustrate these views in direct and indirect ways. The narratives are interwoven with each patient's experience of pain and the fears that acknowledging such pain might interrupt active cancer treatment. Fear of cognitive side effects was prevalent as these individuals strove for greater life expectancy. But as death came closer, pain relief through opioid use was uppermost in their minds.

CONSEQUENCES OF ACKNOWLEDGING UNCONTROLLED PAIN

Vinnie, Connie, and Archie learned that reporting pain to their nurse or doctor sometimes led to undesired consequences. For example, if their physician withheld chemotherapy until the pain was brought under control, they felt they could lose what they considered valuable time. Vinnie chose to tolerate and keep silent about a period of severe pain in order to improve his chances of receiving experimental chemotherapy. This therapy gave him hope for a longer life: "I accepted the pain because I wanted to receive [experimental chemotherapy] ... from Friday to Saturday to Monday I waited because I figured that if they treated me for pain I wouldn't be eligible for the drug."

In a similar vein, Archie thought that to acknowledge the severity of his pain and begin a focused pain management program would be the first step to losing control, no longer being considered a candidate for experimental chemotherapy, and experiencing side effects that could result in him "zonking out." Clarity of mind and involvement with goals and plans were essential features to Archie's sense of self, and he saw his job as achieving pain control in a manner consistent with his goals: "For the last couple of weeks (my goal) has been to manage my pain in such a way that I don't pay the price of total loss ... of my personality ... of myself." Archie felt unprepared for pain management and what he perceived it was costing him:

> I was going to start this new protocol as soon as the radiation side effects wore off, so I was very hopeful ... I was still in control of the situation ... there was no reason for me to believe that I wasn't going to be successful, and if I wasn't something else would be done ... endless possibilities in a way.

But this early sense of endless possibilities was replaced by a perceived loss of control when he started on a focused pain management program: "I didn't appreciate [when] I had to go through pain management that I'd have to make this trade-off and that pain management has such fantastic side effects to it, I didn't know ... the side effects like zonking out, losing your mind."

Archie called this "a trade-off between managing the pain and managing the consequences of managing pain." Pain management with opioids became a burden in of itself because of these side effects. Archie went on to describe how this recognition suddenly dawned on him: "The realization came upon me you know as the weeks went by and all of a sudden it was clear that nobody was going to do anything until the pain was under control ... so that kind of changed priorities and I lost control."

That his disease was rapidly advancing in the setting of rapidly escalating pain, and that many of the changes he was experiencing were associated with progressive disease as well as with opioid side effects, proved difficult for him to countenance. Archie linked focused pain management with deterioration and loss of control because they were occurring simultaneously.

The side effects of opioids and how they affected her quality of life were also of great concern to Connie:

> I don't know how to handle it, you know on the one hand I have less pain with more medicine, on the other hand I'm not quite there, and I guess I prefer to be quite there, you know, because the sleeping is horrible ... I mean basically it's like giving up ... maybe if I'm that sick at some point that I really can't function, well then it's okay, but that's not the case now.

IMPACT OF PAIN ON THE WILL TO LIVE AND DESIRE FOR DEATH

Loss of hope and desire for death followed episodes of severe unrelieved pain for many of these patients. Sometimes a sense of abandonment surfaced in these situations:

> They sent me home from the hospital ... I collapsed and I was in excruciating pain ... they shouldn't have sent me home ... I had no pain control whatsoever ... it was so bad that I would pass out ... they had to bring me back ... dreadful pain control and I wanted to die so badly ... at the end ... I lost hope. (Vinnie)

Vinnie was able to contrast the despair and abandonment he felt when sent home from the hospital with poorly relieved pain and the joy he experienced once the pain was relieved through the use of adequate amounts of opioids: "Once the pain was relieved it was the most beautiful experience of my life, to be able to participate and control the pain." At that time, he spoke of the hope of dying peacefully: "I don't have hope of living, I have hope of dying peacefully and having peace for my family ... so it's a different hope."

Myra's reaction to escalating pain and fear of death also reflected her emotional vulnerability:

> Sometimes I have been known to start yelling that this is horrible, that why don't I just die now ... that it's going to get worse and worse, the pain is going to get worse and worse ... why do I have to live through that until I die? ... I would hope that at that point [with] things getting really bad that I would be under hospice care that has me on a morphine drip, I would hope so ... I mean that's the way it's supposed to happen, at least that's what I've always heard... so that should be what happens and so I shouldn't necessarily have to be in increasing pain till I die.

This statement illustrates the association in Myra's mind between morphine infusions and imminent death; such an association is not uncommon. Pain frequently becomes more severe in the presence of rapidly advancing disease, and parenteral opioids may be necessary to control the pain. In patients' and their family's minds the use of parenteral opioids heralds death, and the two become closely linked. This linkage between opioid infusions and imminent death also emerges in the practice of some clinicians. If a patient is dying in an acute care setting and is without pain or shortness of breath, an opioid infusion may be ordered unrelated to symptoms but solely because the person is near to death, perhaps to ensure that no pain is experienced or to ease the life-to-death transition. However, this practice is not the standard of care in most palliative care settings, where opioids are used in relationship to a symptom.

The fatigue and weariness associated with persistent pain, expressed by many of the patients, were reflected in Connie's words: "There were many times when I was in such pain and such misery I said let me go ... finished, no more of this torture." Connie went on to describe her reason for living and the impact of pain: "I live for joy, I've always done that, what else is there ... if I don't have that I have no reason for living ... so I feel if ever the pain gets to be too much, then somebody's got to help me, I don't want to go on ... but until then, so long as someone can help me with that, I'll live with joy."

Connie spoke of being psychologically ready to die, but her ability to continue her creative work as a photographer made her less inclined to give up hope: "I was ready a long time ago when I was so sick, I said—oh finished—I guess now I'm less ready. You know, when I started to work and the work went fine ... I could be creative again, and now I'm not ready ... but if the pain comes back ... well I don't know."

To be pain free was directly linked in some of the patients' minds to every other aspect of their life. As Harry put it: "No matter what, if I could control the pain I would walk ... I know if I could control the pain I would be, like they say, home free ... when I take care of that pain and I don't have the pain then my mood increases, I would say 90% better." Connie stated: "My moods really depend on how this [leg] feels ... when it feels better I function and when it feels worse I don't. So it's like the physical dictating our moods ... I've always been able to control my moods when I'm able to work and I would get depressed when I can't work and that's really what's happening."

All of the patients expressed similar feelings. Adequate use of opioid drugs to control pain allowed some to reclaim their lives. However, others felt that inadequately managed opioid side effects were depriving them of a meaningful life.

FEAR GENERATED BY UNCONTROLLED PAIN

The fear generated by pain was sometimes related to its perceived meaning, perhaps the implication of disease progression and nearness to death, perhaps the expectation of what the dying process might be like, or perhaps the blackness of the pain experience itself. Vinnie's description of how severe pain blocks out life was graphic:

> Pain is my biggest fear because it blocks out ... it puts me in a darkness and a lack of will to go forward and a desire to die ... the pain wants me to have a vehicle ... just to stop my life. If I could press a button, take a pill, I'd do anything. I just don't want to exist anymore having the pain ... I just want to stop it, I want it to be over with ... the pain has a finality to it that I want to stop right there ... no matter how much good there is left, no matter how much I could enjoy the [rest of my life] ... I wanna go ... I want to be out of this body.

He explained that severe pain trumps the will to live and the ability to find peace. The metaphor could be one of evil winning out over good, or darkness over light, because the negative impact of severe pain is so powerful:

> You can't find [inner peace] in that darkness of pain. ... I can't emphasize that the pain blinds you to all of that, blinds you to all that's positive. I mean the real bad pain ... it just closes you down. You just can't get through it ... it's an iron door and it's one thing you don't wanna go through it; you just wanna, wanna stop.

With Harry, there was a direct association in his mind between increased pain, progression of the disease, and ability to walk. "I got a feeling that [the disease] is getting worse and worse because [of] the pain ... before, I was able to walk." He also expressed dissatisfaction and a certain lack of trust in his pain management approach at home. In the hospital he was pain free, but at home "the pain is getting worse and worse ... they give me a pill; it's supposed to work fast but to me, I don't believe it works that fast ... they are such a small pill ... sometimes I feel like taking the whole bottle."

Myra also expressed fear associated with her escalating pain: "It's very frightening ... I've been very frightened because I'm also in a lot of pain. ... The painkillers stopped working ... I'm worried that it's because the cancer has grown ... so it's a constant reminder." She explained how the persistent pain prevented her from being able to maintain the pretense that everything was all right. "You know it's hard to sit at the dinner table and pretend everything's okay when you are constantly being reminded of the pain ... you know from the pain that everything is far from okay." She went on to say:

The pain makes me worry about dying, because if I'm in pain because the tumor has gotten significantly larger that means I'm losing and the tumor is winning ... but if I'm in pain because simply because the pain med wore off well that's not so scary ... but I don't know which it is ... I just feel I'm beside myself with anxiety.

MEMORIES AND FEARS EVOKED BY THE EXPERIENCE OF SEVERE PAIN

Vinnie and Diana reflected on family members who had experienced pain in their dying. Vinnie's own pain recalled his father's request that he hasten his death. Vinnie felt "too afraid and uncomfortable" to do so, but remained haunted by the experience more than 30 years later: "He had tremendous pain and his pain wasn't well controlled." With Diana, her experience with her father's death three years prior to her own diagnosis with cancer was at first of uncontrolled pain and later well-controlled pain:

At that time if you put a sheet on him he'd scream with pain ... I saw the one extreme where you know, you would think you put a ton of bricks on him by laying a sheet on top of him—to be totally comfortable ... and that's how he spent his last [days], he only lasted about three weeks after that but he was not in excruciating pain, he was very comfortable and he had a peaceful death.

Once a patient had experienced severe pain, fears of that level of pain returning might arise. As Vinnie stated, "Sometimes I get anxiety attacks over it, I don't want ever to go back to being in pain again." The meaning to the patients of poorly controlled or escalating pain was invariably the worsening of the disease and the reality of impending death. Such pain rudely interrupted hopes of "beating this thing" and having a future. Vinnie, talking about going to Cape Cod with his family, explained: "I think I'm thinking a little further ahead, but then when reality strikes with pain ... pain is like a sledgehammer on those thoughts."

CONVERSATIONS WITH GOD AND SELF AROUND PAIN AND THE BREAKING POINT

Unrelieved pain led some of the participants to appeal to God for relief. Harry said: "I ask God, that's the only thing that I want to be pain free ... if I'm going to live for a day or two I just wanna be pain free." For Archie, accepting pain relief measures caused internal conflict and made him question his courage and ability to follow in God's footsteps: "I'm a coward, I, you know, pray to Jesus that I follow him ... in following him you're following sacrifice but yet on the other hand I'm taking pain medicine ... you know I've asked some of the religious people about that and they say don't worry about that."

Connie described suicide as incomprehensible to someone like herself who lived for the joy of life, and if her husband committed suicide after she died as he threatened to do, it would be unforgivable. However, she also gave herself a word of caution: "I may take those words back if ever I cannot for some reason cope with the pain, or misery, or whatever ... I have had times when the pain was such and when my pain medication was not that much under control, and I simply said I don't want to live ... somebody help me out of this."

Universally among these patients, fear of pain (described as shortness of breath by Larry) during the process of dying appeared to be greater than the fear of death or ceasing to exist. Harry expressed the thought in the following terms: "I know we all have to go but the whole thing is the pain. I don't fear to go to sleep and die ... I don't care ... I'd rather die than stay like that, than to be like that in so much pain." Larry also expressed no fear of dying but wanted it to be in a timely and pain-free manner: "I'm going into the great nothingness so that doesn't bother me ... my only question now is to do it in a timely and painless or relatively painless [manner] ... unfortunately I guess with this kind of disease it's almost impossible to knock out the pain."

EFFORTS TO ENSURE A COMFORTABLE DEATH

These seven patients were thinking ahead, trying to come up with strategies to ensure a comfortable death. Larry explained: "You know I've taken great pains up to this stage to, to die as painlessly as possible ... you know I've consciously you know looked into the situation at the hospital." Sometimes, the patients proposed strategies to facilitate a peaceful death. Larry chose a facility he felt would not interfere if he chose to take extra medication: "I didn't think that the doctors would interfere with however I medicated ... if I overmedicated myself that was my business, and their business was that they didn't want any part of that." Myra selected a hospice program because "when things get really bad they crank up whatever they crank up and I find that really reassuring."

INTERPRETING THE MEANING OF PAIN

For all seven patients, the struggle with pain was a dynamic, nonlinear process that was influenced by their appraisal of past experiences with their own pain or that witnessed in others. Other factors included their current medical situation and the pain's meaning within that context, the severity of the immediate pain, the implications of pain management, and thoughts of the future. An internal dialogue typified the struggle as they incorporated new information into their decision-making around pain, its management, and the will to live or desire for death. Past experiences of pain that were remembered as intolerable and terrifying sometimes drove an expressed desire for hastened death. There was no ambivalence or ambiguity, but rather a certainty that death would be the better solution.

In addition to the terror created by the memory of the experience of uncontrolled pain, other issues were central to patients' interpretations of pain. The meaning of a particular pain episode and its possible relationship to the current medical situation, the advancing of the disease process, and the implications for continued existence were all related to these individuals' experience of pain in a fundamental way. These patients were also sensitive to the implications of pain management. They felt that relief of pain was essential, but on the other hand they worried that the use of opioid drugs would detract from their mental clarity, perhaps forcing them to give up awareness and accept somnolence as the price for pain control.

The implications of acknowledging pain when considering further disease-focused treatment protocols was another issue of great importance to these patients. High levels of pain were sometimes tolerated in the hope that another potentially life-prolonging therapy might be offered. Some patients feared that openly expressed pain might have disqualified them from the entry criteria for a new protocol. For these patients the assessment of "total" pain was complex, involving overall suffering, including physical, psychological, social, and spiritual components.

PAIN—A COMMON EXPERIENCE AMONG THOSE LIVING IN THE FACE OF DEATH

Although we have the knowledge and the skill to control most pain, surveys tell us that three-quarters of those with cancer will develop pain at some point during their disease course, and that the severity of their pain will increase as the disease advances (American Pain Society 1999). Half of all adults who die in hospital experience moderate to severe pain in the immediate period before death (SUPPORT Principal Investigators 1995). The fact that pain is part of an individual's disease course should not be a problem in and of itself if it is controlled, but when severe pain is not adequately managed, the human cost can be horrendous, as was clearly described by these seven patients. Pain robbed them of the will to live and destroyed their quality of life. What the disease was not able to destroy in their human spirit, the pain was able to accomplish. For these patients, the experience of pain was a common denominator. Although their pain was adequately controlled most of the time, episodes of severe pain or fear of severe pain made sleep or a hastened death preferable in their minds.

Why do such episodes of severe uncontrolled pain still occur? Is it that we do not yet understand at a very basic level what lies behind the barriers to pain control? The barriers are well known (Jacox 1994), but why do they continue to stand when the human cost is so devastating? The very graphic descriptions of these patients make this cost transparent. Such accounts may lead to a deeper understanding of the reasons why the barriers still stand. Poorly managed cognitive effects of the opioids appeared to be a major reason why these patients were reluctant to use these powerful drugs in adequate amounts to control their pain.

PAIN AND QUALITY OF LIFE

For all these patients, the effects of severe uncontrolled pain were so overwhelming that they dictated every aspect of quality of life. Pain appeared to act as a lightening rod for some, the conspicuous factor that prevented them from being active and living their life. As Harry put it: "If I didn't have the pain I would be home free." For Harry and Connie, pain became a metaphor for all that was wrong. They saw pain as the physical barrier to moving forward in their lives. Vinnie, on the other hand, saw pain as the barrier to his ability to come to terms with his death and teach his family how to "die well." Dying well for Vinnie meant to be pain free, to have his family around him and involved in his personal care, to have no secrets about his illness and closeness to death, and to experience peace of mind, knowing that his family was prepared for his death. The grief they would suffer would be a "healing grief." The effective use of opioid drugs was critical for this "good death" to occur.

The importance of good pain management is evident in studies asking terminally ill patients to identify domains of quality end-of-life care. In a cross-sectional, stratified random national survey to determine factors considered important at the end of life by patients ($n = 340$), their family members ($n =$

332), physicians ($n = 361$), and other care providers ($n = 429$), management of pain and other symptoms was ranked as important by more than 70% of respondents across all groups. Participants ranked freedom from pain as the factor of most importance to them (Steinhauser et al. 2000). The seven patients who took part in the investigation by Coyle (unpublished manuscript) clearly reveal the reasons why freedom from pain, or control of pain, can have such significance to respondents in this and similar studies. The human dimensions of uncontrolled pain not only to the individual experiencing it but to family and staff, the starkness of severe pain and the associated loss of autonomy, the dependency on the skills, knowledge, and attitudes of others for relief of pain, and the vulnerability of everyone involved make it a constant source of wonder to me that episodes of severe, uncontrolled pain are still such a common experience among advanced cancer patients, even in the most sophisticated institutions. Some of the narratives give a glimpse from the participant's perspective into why this may be happening.

TAKING CONTROL—PAIN MANAGEMENT TRADE-OFFS

Across the board, the participants in the study by Coyle (unpublished manuscript) were actively involved in their pain management decisions and carefully weighed the benefit versus burden of the use of escalating doses of opioid drugs. They considered the meaning of the pain, the implications of acknowledging uncontrolled pain, and how pain management might affect their goals.

The balance between pain control and side effects from opioid use presented Archie and Connie with a difficult situation. Both of their concerns about opioid side effects, and Archie's worry that emphasis on pain control would mean de-emphasis of disease control, are recognized in the general pain literature as patient-related barriers to cancer pain management (Jacox 1994). Archie's experience clearly illustrates the fears of some advanced cancer patients. When pain management became the focus of his care, disease control was no longer at the forefront. Archie equated pain management with loss of control—that was his experience and he described it most eloquently.

For Connie, the sedative and cognitive side effects of the opioid drugs ("not being quite there") were initially unacceptable to her as she strove to live a meaningful and productive life and to continue her photography. She opted to tolerate a higher level of pain in order to be "quite there" and awake and alert. When she was unable to get out of her chair because of the severity of her movement-related pain, the trade-off was no longer worth it to her. The quality of her life had diminished and she desired only sleep to escape from the pain and loss of meaning.

Bruera and colleagues (1989) conducted a prospective study to examine the cognitive effects of opioid administration in patients with cancer pain admitted to a palliative care unit. Forty consecutive patients with cancer pain receiving intermittent opioids were admitted to the study. Twenty patients had undergone no change in opioid dose or type in the previous week, and the others had received an increase of at least 30% no more than 3 days before. The results suggested that patients whose opioid dose was increased significantly experience significant cognitive impairment (increased somnolence and sedation), but that these effects disappear after approximately 1 week. Unfortunately, in the Coyle study both Connie and Archie continued to experience cognitive side effects from the level of opioid drugs they needed to control their pain, despite opioid rotation, changes in the route of drug administration, adjuvant drugs, and the use of psychostimulants.

Quantitative measures are important tools by which to assess pain severity and pain relief. But unless the human dimensions are recognized—demoralization, a sense of hopelessness, defeat, and deep-seated fatigue, and yet the fear that the measures that can bring them most relief, the opioid drugs, will deprive them of their mental clarity, the last bastion of human dignity—then episodes of uncontrolled pain will in all probability remain the lot of many of those living and dying with advanced cancer. The participants in the Coyle study have performed a great service by revealing the human experience of severe, uncontrolled pain in all of its starkness. They also shed light not only on the power of the opioid drugs to bring them relief but also on the deleterious effect of inadequately managed side effects on their well-being.

REFERENCES

American Pain Society. *Principles of Analgesic Use with Treatment of Acute Pain and Cancer Pain,* 4th ed. Glenview, IL: American Pain Society, 1999.

Anderson KO, Mendoza, TR, Valero V, et al. Minority cancer patients and their providers: pain management attitudes and practice. *Cancer* 2000; 88:1929–1938.

Anderson KO, Richman SP, Hurley J, et al. Cancer pain management among underserved minority outpatients: perceived needs and barriers to optimal control. *Cancer* 2002; 94:2295–2304.

Bookbinder M, Coyle N, Kiss M, et al. Implementing national standards for cancer pain management: program model and evaluation. *J Pain Symptom Manage* 1995; 12:334–347.

Bruera E, Macmillan K, Hanson J, MacDonald RN. The cognitive effects of the administration of narcotic analgesics in patients with cancer pain. *Pain* 1989; 39:13–16.

Brescia F, Portenoy RK, Ryan M, Drasnoff L, Gray G. Pain, opioid use and survival in hospitalized patients with advanced cancer. *J Clin Oncol* 1992; 10:149–155.

Cherny N, Catane R. Professional negligence in the management of cancer pain. *Cancer* 1995; 76:2181–2184.

Cherny N, Coyle N. Suffering in the advanced cancer patient: a definition and taxonomy. *J Palliat Care* 1994;10:57–70.

Cherny N, Portenoy NK. Practical issues in the management of cancer pain. In: Wall PD, Melzack R (Eds). *Textbook of Pain*, 3rd ed. Edinburgh: Churchill Livingstone, 1994, pp 1437–1467.

Cleeland CS, Gonin R, Hatfield AK, et al. Pain and its treatment in outpatients with metastatic cancer. *N Engl J Med* 1994; 330:592–596.

Coyle N. Facilitating pain management in the home: opioid related issues. C*urr Pain Headache Rep* 2001; 5:217–226.

Daut RC, Cleeland CS. The prevalence and severity of pain in cancer. *Cancer* 1982; 50:1913–1918.

Fishman B. The treatment of suffering in patients with cancer pain: cognitive behavioral approaches. In: Foley KM, Bonica JJ, Ventafridda V (Eds). *Proceedings of the Second International Congress on Cancer Pain,* Advances in Pain Research and Therapy, Vol. 16. New York: Raven Press, 1991, pp 301–316.

Foley KM. The relationship of pain and symptom management to patient requests for physician-assisted suicide. *J Pain Symptom Manage* 1991; 6:289–297.

Gonzales GR, Coyle N. Treatment of cancer pain in a former opioid abuser: fears of the patient and staff and their influence on care. *J Pain Symptom Manage* 1992; 7:246–249.

Grossman SA, Shiedler VR, Swedeen K, Mucenski J, Piantadosi S. Correlations of patient and caregiver ratings of cancer pain. *J Pain Symptom Manage* 1991; 6:53–57.

Gunnarsdottir S, Donovan HS, Serlin RC, Voge C, Ward S. Patient-related barriers to pain management: the barriers questionnaire. *Pain* 2002; 99:385–396.

Institute of Medicine. *Approaching Death: Assessing Care at the End of Life*. Washington, DC: National Academy Press, 1997, p 5.

Jacox A, Carr DB, Payne R. *Management of Cancer Pain.* Clinical Practice Guidelines No. 9, AHCPR Publication No. 94-0592. Rockville, MD: U.S. Department for Health and Human Services, Public Health Service, Agency for Health Care Policy and Research, 1994.

Joint Commission on Accreditation of Healthcare Organizations. *Pain Assessment and Management: an Organizational Approach,* 2000. Available via the Internet: www.jcaho.org.

Joranson DE, Cleeland CS, Weisman DE. Opioids in chronic pain and non-cancer pain: a survey of state medical board members. *Fed Bull: J Med Licensure Discipline* 1992; 79:15–49.

Kanner R, Portenoy RK. Unavailability of narcotic analgesics for ambulatory cancer patients in New York City. *J Pain Symptom Manage* 1986; 1:187–189.

Levin DN, Cleeland CS, Dar R. Public attitudes towards cancer pain. *Cancer* 1985; 63:2328–2335.

Morrison RS, Wallenstein S, Natale DK, Senzel RS, Huang LL. "We don't carry that"—failure of pharmacies in predominantly nonwhite neighborhoods to stock opioid analgesics. *N Engl J Med* 2001; 342:1023–1026.

Ng K, von Gunten CF. Symptoms and attitudes of 100 consecutive patients admitted to an acute hospice/palliative care unit. *J Pain Symptom Manage* 1998; 16:307–316.

Pargeon KL, Hailey BJ. Barriers to effective pain management: a review of the literature. *J Pain Symptom Manage* 1999; 18:358–368.

Resnik DB. Stocking opioids in community pharmacies. *J Pain Symptom Manage* 2001; 22(1):537–538.

Steinhauser KE, Christakis NA, Clipp EC, et al. Factors considered important at the end of life by patients, family, physicians, and other care providers. *JAMA* 2000; 284:2476–2482.

SUPPORT Principal Investigators. A controlled trial to improve care for seriously ill hospitalized patients. The study to understand prognoses and preferences for outcomes and risks of treatments (SUPPORT). *JAMA* 1995; 274:1591–1598.

Taylor EJ, Ferrell BR, Grant M, Cheyney L. Managing cancer pain at home: the decisions and ethical conflicts of patients, family caregivers and homecare nurses. *Oncol Nurs Forum* 1993; 20:919–927.

Von Roenn JH, Cleeland CS, Gonin R, Hatfield AK, Pandya KJ. Physician attitudes and practice in cancer pain management: a survey from the Eastern Cooperative Oncology Group. *Ann Intern Med* 1993;119:121–126.

Wallace K, Reade B, Pasera C, Olson G. Staff nurses' perception of barriers to effective pain management. *J Pain Symptom Manage* 1995; 10:204–213.

Ward SE, Berry PE, Misiewicz H. Concerns about analgesics among patients and family caregivers in a hospice setting. *Res Nurs Health* 1996; 19:205–211.

Correspondence to: Nessa Coyle, PhD, NP, FAAN, Department of Neurology and Pain Service, Memorial-Sloan-Kettering Cancer Center, 1275 York Avenue, New York, NY 10021, USA. Email: coylen@mskcc.org.

Opioids and Pain Relief: A Historical Perspective,
Progress in Pain Research and Management, Vol.
25, edited by Marcia L. Meldrum, IASP Press,
Seattle, © 2003.

14

The Property of Euphoria: Research and the Cancer Patient

Marcia L. Meldrum

*John C. Liebeskind History of Pain Collection, Louise M. Darling Biomedical
Library, and Department of History, University of California, Los Angeles,
Los Angeles, California, USA*

When the patient comes to the physician with her story and symptoms, the physician's response draws on his knowledge of science, his clinical experience, and his reading of the literature, but also on his imagined narrative of the patient, of her pain and its treatment, and of her response to treatment, a narrative that, as Martha Stoddard Holmes (this volume) has written, is culturally and historically specific. Nowhere is this more true than when the physician is considering a prescription of opiates for a patient in severe chronic pain. (This chapter will use "opiates" to refer to the drugs themselves, as was the usage during most of the period under discussion.) In the 21st century, we see opium and its relatives through the prism of many histories and mythologies, several of them described by the authors in this book. My endeavor in this chapter is to consider how the World Health Organization (WHO) analgesic ladder represents a rewriting of the cultural narrative of opiate use and to what extent it has changed the imagined narrative in the minds of American physicians and their patients.

As Caroline Acker (this volume) has discussed, the original legislation regulating opiate prescriptions in the United States, the Harrison Narcotic Act of 1914, represented the intersection of a number of currents in American reform; prominent among these was the Progressive drive to impose order and morality on the growing immigrant working class. The Progressives' faith in the power of scientific data and method to provide solutions to social problems strengthened and informed their certainty of moral rectitude. Manifestations of these Progressivist convictions included the American Medical Association's Council on Pharmacy and Chemistry, established in 1903 to provide physicians with scientific information on the composition and efficacy of the plethora of patent medicines on the market; the Eighteenth Amendment's constitutional prohibition of the manufacture and sale of alcohol; and the Bureau of Social Hygiene's Committee on Drug Addiction and its offshoot and namesake, the National Research Council (NRC)'s Committee on Drug Addiction, organized in 1928–1929 to identify an effective non-narcotic analgesic.

Physicians' support of the Harrison Act reflected their participation in Progressivist ideals and their interest in the professionalization of medicine. Morphine, laudanum, and cocaine had long been useful tools for the practitioner, but they had acquired connotations of quackery as well, through their use as the chief ingredient in many patent medicines of dubious value. As evidence gathered in the early 1900s of iatrogenic dependence and of diversion to the illicit market, even responsible medical use of the opiate drugs suggested associations with the dark and hopeless figure of the addict. Physicians preferred to be associated with the white coat of the surgeon and the scientist, and with the new drugs emerging from the research laboratory—aspirin, salvarsan, thyroxin, insulin, and the new antitoxins. Using the methods of Paul Ehrlich and Torald Sollman, the NRC researchers' disciplined program would, it was hoped, develop a powerful new analgesic, one free of overtones of hucksterism and crime. Until that day, the opiates could be used, but with restraint, as the new legislation mandated. Morphine could be used, along with derivatives such as meperidine, but the rapid action of heroin made it more dangerous to the patient, as well as more attractive to the illicit user. In 1949, WHO began a concerted and largely successful effort to encourage all countries to ban the medicinal use of heroin (World Health Organization 1950).

PRESCRIPTIONS AND PRACTICE: 1950–1979

How did opiate practice develop, with restraint, over the 50 years between 1929 and 1979? What guidelines for use did the experts offer in the standard texts consulted by physicians? In examining these texts, the reader will quickly identify the issues considered salient: levels of dosage; scheduling of doses—p.r.n. ("as the occasion arises") or at scheduled intervals ("by the clock"); the risk of tolerance—as the patient's system adjusts to the drug, larger doses may be required to produce the same analgesic effect; and, of course, the risk of addiction.

The most comprehensive discussion of all issues of pain and analgesia in this period came from the pen of John Bonica (1917–1994), whose great work, *The Management of Pain*, first appeared in 1953. His perspective on the use of opiates in medicine and the risk of iatrogenic addiction is characteristically level-headed. "The *effects* of opiate addiction are few as long as the drug is taken. Ill health, … crime and degeneracy are the result, not of the pharmacological effects of morphine, but of the sacrifice of food, money, social position, and self-respect in order to buy the daily dose of the drug" (Bonica 1953).

Bonica urged that the practitioner be prudent, but attentive to his patient's distress, in prescribing. He urged the physician to titrate dosage by "the intensity of pain … the most important factor determining the amount of analgesic medication needed." However, he maintained that opiates should be "reserved until the non-narcotic analgesics no longer afford relief" and then given "in optimal doses … the smallest amount that will cause the desired effects." Oral morphine (considered less potent, so that larger doses would be needed than with the injected drug) is "reserved for chronic pain such as occurs with cancer, when repeated doses at more or less regular intervals are necessary." In the last days of life, he wrote, the patient's comfort was the predominant concern: "the analgesia, euphoria, and tranquillity afforded by the wise use of narcotics are a blessing to the patient and his family, and the final weeks are made easy and comfortable, justifying the inevitable addiction" (Bonica 1953).

There is no suggestion here that the physician should avoid large doses or regular doses if needed to relieve pain. Bonica saw dosage by the clock "at more or less regular intervals" as necessary in chronic pain, and he did not limit this practice to cancer or to dying patients. He considered tolerance to be unavoidable, thus the need for starting at the lowest dose. Addiction too was inevitable, but he clearly differentiated medical dependence from the desperation of the street addict (Bonica 1953).

As Bonica himself often noted, only in rare cases did writers of texts on cancer or other painful diseases devote more than a few lines to the problem of pain relief. In 1956, however, a small volume appeared on *The Management of Pain in Cancer,* edited by M.J. Schiffrin, an Illinois anesthesiologist. In the preface, Warren Cole, head of surgery at the University of Illinois, explained the dilemma physicians often faced and the unspoken fear that troubled them:

> We must appreciate that severe constant pain will destroy the morale of the sturdiest individual. … On many occasions the terminal phase progresses so rapidly that there is not enough time, between onset of the severe pain and death, for addiction to become very important. … But since it is … impossible to predict duration of life with cancer, we are often loathe to give liberal amounts of narcotics because the drug addiction itself may become a hideous spectacle. (Cole 1956)

The book's single chapter on opiate drugs, written by Schiffrin and E.J. Gross, a pharmacologist, echoed Bonica's recommendations: "If the prognosis indicates a terminal course that can be measured in weeks, every effort should be made to provide relief of pain regardless of ... [the risk of] addiction. ... The medical and social problems of addiction are unimportant when the few remaining days of life need the blessed relief provided by the opiates." But, in the case of a longer prognosis, "addiction and particularly tolerance are important in the patient with long term chronic pain. In such instances every effort should be made to put off the use of the potent addicting drugs until all other measures have been exhausted."

When the patient's pain warranted the use of opiates, however, the physician should prescribe adequate doses "promptly on the appearance of pain. Pain itself is a most potent antagonist to the drug. ... Therefore, full doses should be given when the pain is moderate instead of waiting until the patient writhes in pain." The authors cautioned against by-the-clock dosage, as the patient might be undermedicated: "Addicting analgesics are to be ordered on the basis of pain, not according to the clock or nursing habits" (Schiffrin and Gross 1956).

Nursing texts echoed these themes. In their 1972 text, *Nursing Care of the Cancer Patient,* Rosemary Bouchard and Norma Owens discussed pain briefly in a single chapter:

> Only when obstruction of an organ ... and bone or nerve involvement occur does the patient with cancer actually experience pain [which can usually be treated with aspirin and other non-opiate drugs]. ... Once narcotics are started, both the nurse and the physician must constantly assess the degree of pain the patient is experiencing before administering these drugs in order to minimize the development of tolerance or addiction. ... [The nurse may provide psychological support and comfort measures to reduce the patient's need for strong narcotics.] It should be emphasized, however, that medication should not be withheld when the patient really needs it to alleviate his pain since [in advanced and terminal cases] there is no chance for cure or rehabilitation. (Bouchard and Owens 1972)

The texts that were available to the practitioner in the 1950s and 1960s, therefore, did not suggest that he should avoid using opiate drugs or limit the amounts given, but that he should carefully titrate the dosage to relieve even moderate pain in painful chronic diseases such as cancer. There was some disagreement on the scheduling of doses and the appropriate use of opiates before the prognosis could be "measured in weeks." Once death was near, all writers agreed that the physician should not hesitate to prescribe the powerful pain drugs. But Cole's warning of the "hideous spectacle" of an addicted patient living for months, or even years, suggests a vivid cultural image that must have haunted many physicians as they reached for the triplicate prescription forms.

But what occurred in practice? Did physicians follow the advice of Bonica or the more conservative recommendations of Schiffrin and Gross? Or were tacit rules followed in hospitals that residents and student nurses learned through observation of their seniors? There is little in the way of systematic evidence. In order to understand what happened in practice, the historian must search through a variety of sources to try to find first-hand accounts by observers with different perspectives.

Bonica himself commented: "The attitude and practice of some physicians to prescribe narcotics in excessive doses as soon as the diagnosis of inoperability is made 'because the end is inevitable and the patient should be made as comfortable as possible' denotes a lack of understanding"; he suggested that this practice often led to "unnecessarily premature addiction" (Bonica 1953).

A chaplain who shared the last days of 20 patients dying from cancer wrote of his experience in the *Journal of Pastoral Care*:

> Only two of the 20 patients were really permitted to *meet* death … several had such terrible pain that extremely heavy sedation had to be given; but the others were drugged into lethargy as the time drew near, well before they had lost their wits, so that they had no opportunity to know that they were going. Doctors avoided the subject of death, maintained with the patients the fiction that they were going to get better, did not let them knowingly meet the last great experience of life. (Reeves 1960)

A nurse studying for an anthropology degree conducted observations on a cancer ward in a hospital (not one she had worked in herself). She wrote this account of a patient whose doctor sharply increased his morphine dose as death neared:

> Mr. Piel … was semicomatose, but moaning with pain from several pathologic fractures. … Dr. Long told Annette [the patient's nurse] to increase Mr. Piel's morphine to 60 mg. every two hours. Annette looked at Dr. Long and repeated the dose, and Dr. Long confirmed it. Later … Annette said [to the observer] "in nursing school … we were taught that 15 mg. was the maximum dose to be given at any one time. I know he's been on a gradually increasing dose, but I still remember that earlier learning." "Was the medication given as ordered?" "Oh yes … He had two doses." The patient was given the prescribed amount twice and died before the next scheduled dose (German 1979).

(The pseudonyms in this account were assigned by German.) Fifteen milli-
grams was the "customary maximum dose" cited in many texts (Nealon 1965).

The observing nurse recorded another incident on the ward, when, at
four in the afternoon, a newly admitted patient "shouted out from her room,
'I have a lot of pain, and I need something for it.'" The nurse told her that
she would have to wait and talk to the doctor "when he comes in. ... You
were given something at three o'clock, and you only have an order for every
four hours" (German 1979).

The nurse-educator and pain specialist Ada Jacox described her observations of nursing practices with opiates in her 1977 text on pain:

> They show this concern [about addiction] by withholding medication
> because it is still "one-half to three-fourths of an hour early" before the
> four-hour interval between dosages expires. It seems paradoxical to think
> that nothing is done about the fact that the medication is not lasting the time
> interval indicated by the doctor's orders. Instead of evaluating the effec-
> tiveness of the current dosage and frequency, the battle goes on repeatedly
> with the patient complaining of pain two or three hours before the
> medication is given and the nurse insisting that the patient must wait. The
> patient becomes more irritable and anxious as his pain increases; mean-
> while, the nurse becomes impatient and begins to believe that the patient
> ... is addicted to his medication. ... The drama is absurd. (Jacox 1977)

Finally, a systematic study, small but disturbing, was conducted by
Richard Marks and Edward Sachar at Montefiore Hospital in the early 1970s.
(A similar study conducted in British hospitals is reported by Hunt et al.
[1977]). Marks and Sachar gathered data on opiate prescriptions, dosages
actually given, and "distress" scores reported by 37 inpatients in structured
interviews. All of the patients had diseases or injuries for which pain is a
well-recognized symptom. Most were receiving meperidine, with varying
dosage levels prescribed every four hours "p.r.n." (Two patients were receiving morphine, but the authors converted the amounts to equivalent meperidine dosage for purposes of comparison; 100 mg of meperidine is considered equivalent to 15 mg of morphine.) The dosages prescribed by the house
physicians were not well correlated to the pain and distress levels the patients reported to Marks and Sachar; however, whatever the dosage, the
authors found that these patients received only 25–50% of the prescribed
amounts. The average prescription for the 12 patients who reported "marked
distress" was 66 mg every 4 hours (a maximum of 396 mg a day); the average
dosage these patients received was 103 mg/day, slightly more than a quarter
of the amount allowed by the house staff. The average dosage received by

the 15 patients who reported "moderate distress" was only 72 mg/day. Twenty-three patients reported that their pain and distress often returned between scheduled doses (Marks and Sachar 1973).

Based on their follow-up interviews with the house staff, the authors cited the residents' lack of knowledge about the opiates and their misconceptions about the dangers of addiction as the major reasons for the undermedication. Other reasons identified were the nurses' interpretation of "p.r.n." orders, residents' and nurses' fears of errors and overmedication, and their "puritanical counter-reactions" to drugs that seemed to cause euphoric reactions in patients. The overall tendency was to use the opiates as sparingly as possible. Marks and Sachar suggested in conclusion that "for many physicians these drugs may have a special emotional significance that interferes with their rational use" (Marks and Sachar 1973).

From these first-hand observations, we may draw some inferences about how opiates were used to alleviate pain, particularly cancer pain, in some, or perhaps most, American hospitals, between 1950 and 1979. There was a distinct division between patients receiving curative treatment and those acknowledged to be dying. Both physicians and nurses tended to administer these drugs sparingly while the patient was receiving curative treatment. They cited the standard or maximum dosage as 15 mg of morphine or its equivalent. Nurses might interpret "by-the-clock" prescriptions as a way to ration opiate use or understand "p.r.n." as an indication for minimal medication. However, when the physician determined that the patient's condition was terminal, with only a short time to live, he or she was likely to increase the dosage, in some cases to very high levels; many patients were thus heavily sedated or comatose in the days or hours before death.

Both texts and practice observations convey a level of discomfort with opiates that was apparently due more to the drugs' "special emotional significance" than to an informed understanding of their pharmacology. This unease was not purely the fear of addiction: most of the physicians interviewed by Marks and Sachar (1973) stated their belief that fewer than 5% of drug addicts began their habit in a medical setting. I suggest that it was a more nebulous but very real characteristic of the opiates, and their effect on patient behavior, that troubled the prescribing physician and the dispensing nurse: the property of euphoria.

THE PROPERTY OF EUPHORIA

"A feeling of well being that has an exhilarating quality," as Bonica described it, was a well-recognized effect of taking morphine or another opiate (Bonica 1953). Schiffrin and Gross (1956) described this as a positive factor:

> Morphine often produces a sense of well-being beyond what might be expected to occur on the basis of the reaction to the relief of pain. This sense of well-being is a desirable effect because the patient is comfortable and cooperative. ... The patient is aware of pain, but he feels that it is no longer part of him. He recognizes it as he would an impersonal object in the room; and since his thoughts are no longer completely centered on pain, he can think and act in a rational manner. ... The picture is completely different when *euphoria* results from the administration of a drug such as morphine; then the patient is definitely uncooperative, and his thoughts are turned inward as he experiences a sense of exhilaration and exaltation. ... The patient's response to euphoria ... will warn of the impending danger of addiction." (Schiffrin and Gross 1956; emphasis added)

"Euphoria," as opposed to "well-being," they suggested, was an undesirable effect of opiates in certain patients, to be recognized by the patient's exhilaration and failure to act rationally, that is, to be cooperative with the doctor or nurse. It seems probable that the difference between euphoria and well-being was often hard to differentiate, and that clinicians anxious about addiction might readily misinterpret the behavior of patients receiving opiates for pain.

As Raymond Houde, a leading American researcher on analgesic drugs, commented in 1978:

> Ironically, the capacity to induce a sense of well-being, or euphoria, is a property of the narcotics which we have been making a great effort to eliminate from the so-called "ideal analgesic" of our aspirations. This unfortunate paradox has been the result of an association of euphoria with drug abuse and with the popular misconception that drugs with this capability enslave, demoralize, and lead the unwitting patient down the primrose path to addiction.

He added drily, "We have not seen any outward signs of elation in our cancer patients receiving on-demand narcotics" (Houde 1979).

The imagined story of the opiate drugs in 1970s America, the drama unfolding in the mind of the physician, the nurse, and the patient, was in part about the fear of addiction, but I suggest that fear was only the most clearly defined theme in a complex and emotionally resonant narrative. Morphine and its cousins were implicitly associated in the cultural consciousness with the loss of rationality and responsibility, with a euphoric state unrelated to the realities of disease and treatment. Further, because of the medical practices linking unrestricted use to the final days, the drugs were closely associated with the inevitable approach of death. To take opiates, therefore, in our unspoken beliefs, was to be less than rational, less than living—to lose control and perhaps to lose selfhood. It was to pass through an unseen boundary into the wasteland of the cancer victim, the out-of-control, the hopelessly ill, the dying. It was not what the patient wished to be given or what the caregiver wished to administer. I have written here in the past tense, but this narrative continues to resonate in the 21st century.

ALTERNATIVE NARRATIVE: SLOAN-KETTERING

But an alternative narrative has taken shape. In the late 1970s and 1980s, two clinical research programs established the basis for the WHO cancer pain relief program and for the rewriting of the standard texts, at least on the management of cancer pain (Swerdlow, this volume). The work of Raymond Houde and Ada Rogers at Sloan-Kettering in New York, and of Cicely Saunders and Robert Twycross at St. Christopher's Hospice in London, re-established the opiates as an important part of medical science and questioned the presumed inevitable association with addiction and loss of selfhood. Their approaches and methods were very different, and their meetings at the first international conferences on cancer pain were indeed somewhat acrimonious.

Houde's research was part of the NRC Committee on Drug Addiction's project to identify the effective non-narcotic analgesic. By the late 1940s, researchers had found a number of experimental compounds, variations of the morphine molecule, ready to be evaluated for analgesic efficacy on clinical patients. The committee drafted the young internist Houde and sent him to Michigan to study pharmacology with Maurice Seevers and then to the Addiction Research Center in Lexington, Kentucky, to learn about addiction. In 1951, he hired a research nurse, Ada Rogers, and a psychologist, Stanley Wallenstein, and started work at James Ewing Hospital, part of the Memorial-Sloan-Kettering complex. Over the next 20 years, Houde and Rogers conducted thousands of analgesic trials, comparing new drugs with a standard medication, usually morphine. Although their methods set a standard in the field, they enjoyed limited recognition because their results, regularly reported to the Committee on Drug Addiction, were rarely published in the general medical literature (Modell and Houde 1958; Houde 1995; Rogers 1995). (Howard Thaler, a pharmacologist at Sloan-Kettering, is currently working on an database and analysis of Houde's more than 17,000 studies.)

The patients Houde and Rogers recruited for their studies were poor and working-class New Yorkers, in advanced or terminal stages of cancer, many without hope of cure. They lay in their hospital beds for weeks or months, often until they died. When Rogers arrived with her "little basket" of coded vials and asked them to participate in a pain study, there was an opportunity to participate in something worthwhile. "Soon the word got around," she recalled, and people "were very good about going on study." Rogers visited her study patients every hour and asked about their degree of pain. She was at the hospital for 10 hours a day, and often longer, if one of her charges was having trouble with nausea or sedation. Few patients in any hospital would have received such a level of personalized attention and care (Rogers 1995).

She never knew exactly what she was giving them in the coded vials. Houde's research strategy was based on the concept that the patients would give you an accurate, objective report if you defined their choices clearly and removed any possibility of bias. He adapted the idea of double-blinding from Harry Gold at Cornell. From Henry Beecher at Harvard, and from his own experiments with student volunteers at Michigan, he had learned that any individual's perception of pain was complicated by multiple variables— including his or her emotional state, expectations or fears for the future, previous medications or treatments, and the course of the disease itself. "I have no way of knowing actually what these people are feeling," he rea- soned. "So the only thing I can do is to have them serve as their own control, and use some kind of standard which I can compare it to" (Houde 1995).

Houde made each patient his or her "own control" with a crossover study design, in which the patient received a series of graded doses of a test medication, randomized against graded doses of a known standard drug— morphine or aspirin. The "double dummy" series would test the drug in both oral and parenteral forms against a standard drug or placebo, also given by both routes. The test or "challenge" doses were given once a day; the rest of the time, the patients remained on their regular prescriptions from the house staff. On Rogers' visits, she asked for their report about their level of pain— none, slight, moderate, severe; about their level of relief on a similar four- or five-point scale; about side effects. And she added her own observations. If a patient was in even moderate pain after receiving one of her doses, she was ready to provide rescue medication with a known drug. The data from multiple test series conducted on multiple patients, calculated and analyzed, gave very precise information about *relative* degrees of analgesia, relative duration of relief, relative levels of side effects such as nausea and respira- tory depression, and the relative development of tolerance to all these. Houde explained: "We sought out a balance between a drug's good effects and its bad effects ... the only way we could determine that, of course, was in relative terms" (Houde 1995; Rogers 1995).

The patient population at Ewing gradually changed, as radiation treatments and chemotherapy drugs were introduced. Hospital stays became much shorter, and patients receiving other investigational treatments were not available to Houde for analgesic studies. By the early 1970s, most of his projects were single-dose comparisons in postoperative patients. But he and Rogers were much in demand to advise on difficult pain management cases in all wards of the hospital. They applied a patient-centered philosophy, relating each patient's variable needs to what they had learned about the good and bad effects of each drug: "Each particular patient presents a problem which should be approached in an individual way in proper evaluation and treatment." "The patient expects to be treated as a whole human being. ... Our aim for the patient who has advanced cancer is an understanding of his suffering and, through understanding, relief" (Rogers 1979; Houde 1995). Memorial-Sloan-Kettering approved the formation of a Pain Consult Service and the creation of a Training Fellowship in 1971, enabling Houde and Rogers to disseminate their findings and ideas to other clinicians. Among the Fellows trained in the Pain Service in the 1970s and 1980s were Kathleen Foley, Ronald Kanner, Russell Portenoy, and Richard Payne.

ALTERNATIVE NARRATIVE: ST. CHRISTOPHER'S HOSPICE

Cicely Saunders' research program at her model hospice in East London approached the problem of analgesic efficacy from a different perspective (Clark, this volume; Faull and Nicholson, this volume). The patients had various illnesses and came from all walks of life, but all were presumed to be near the end of life. Saunders' goal was to identify, and to demonstrate with evidence, the most effective methods of maintaining the patients' well-being and of helping them to find personal meaning as death approached. As she has stated, "They are challenged to meet adversity and the achievement must be theirs, not ours. ... Okay, you control pain, you control the other symptoms. ... [but] your ultimate aim is not just to see the pain gone, but to see a patient free of pain doing something" (Saunders 1993). When Robert Twycross began his comparison studies at St. Christopher's in 1971, he used a crossover model similar to that employed by Houde, but within the very different context of regular by-the-clock administration and "total care" that constituted standard hospice practice. He demonstrated that, within this setting, oral morphine was as effective as diamorphine and more reliable than the Brompton cocktail; he showed also that patient tolerance and dependence on opiates were not inevitable with prolonged use and were manageable clinical problems when they did occur (Twycross 1977, 1979a,b; Clark, this volume; Faull and Nicholson, this volume).

The first event to bring the New York and London researchers together was a one-day special session on cancer pain at the First World Congress on Pain in 1975; this was the meeting at which Twycross, in his own description, "strode to the podium" with his British colleagues cheering him on, to challenge Houde's conclusions (Faull and Nicholson, this volume). The discussion continued at the First International Symposium on Pain in Advanced Cancer in Venice in 1978, at the Symposium on the Treatment of Cancer and Postoperative Pain organized by the Swedish Academy of Sciences in 1981, and at the WHO Consultation on the Cancer Pain Relief Program in 1982 (Swerdlow, this volume). Despite their common interest in cancer pain relief and similar comparison methodologies, the Sloan-Kettering and St. Christopher's groups had very different objectives and interpreted their findings from widely divergent perspectives.

Ostensibly, the main points of dispute were the potency of oral morphine relative to parenteral morphine, the use of by-the-clock versus p.r.n. administration, and the inevitability of tolerance. Houde's objective was the precise differentiation of available analgesics, and he addressed these questions from that perspective. He had measured the analgesic effects of a single isolated dose of oral morphine versus a single isolated dose of the injected drug. He had compared and quantified the degree of tolerance to be expected with prolonged use of each particular opiate medication. Although he and Rogers gave medication for even moderate degrees of pain—"I didn't want to force the patient to say they had severe pain or they wouldn't get medication," Houde (1995) has explained—they needed to make a quantitative comparison between the patient's pain before and after each test dose. A "regular giving" regimen whereby the patient was maintained in a steady analgesic state and never allowed to experience more than slight pain would have invalidated the protocol.

Twycross's objective was the maintenance of patient well-being throughout the hospice stay. The outcome measures were not precise differentials, but overall levels of analgesia and well-being. Oral morphine had clear advantages in terms of patient comfort and autonomy; in the context of regular by-the-clock dosage, which also contributes to patient well-being, the oral drug provided a consistent level of effective relief. Tolerance was unlikely to develop if the patient was maintained on adequate dosage; if it did develop, it could be managed without compromising pain relief. The risk of tolerance, however measured, was not a sufficient reason for minimizing dosage.

Despite their divergent objectives and interests, which often prompted public debates, the two groups agreed in more ways than they disagreed, as illustrated in the following passages from the papers presented at the Venice Symposium. On dosage levels, for example, Houde stated: "It is better to be governed by the demands of the particular clinical situation than by dogma." And Twycross said that "the right dose of any analgesic is that which gives adequate relief. ... Pain unrelieved by other measures, not short life-expectancy, is the primary criterion for prescription of morphine or other narcotic analgesics."

On by-the-clock administration, Twycross cautioned: "To allow pain to re-emerge before administering the next dose not only causes unnecessary suffering but encourages tolerance." And Houde responded:

> We have little reason to doubt this from our observations, since the more severe the pain is allowed to become, the more difficult it seems to be to control. ... [T]he on-demand prescription forces the patient to re-experience pain before taking or requesting medication, which can be very damaging to the morale of many patients.

However, he cautioned that the "regular giving" method could mask the development of new painful complications in the disease, or an unpredictable remission and decrease in pain intensity.

Finally, Twycross stated repeatedly: "Tolerance is usually not a practical problem." Houde's view was that tolerance and physical dependence "are properties of narcotics. They are not important if you adjust your doses. Remember that though patients can gain tolerance and physical dependence, they can also lose it" (Houde 1979; Twycross 1979a,b).

On certain critical points, then, the Sloan-Kettering group and the St. Christopher's group were very much in agreement. Both had identified morphine as the most reliable drug, despite the availability of many other analgesics (diamorphine, meperidine, metopon, methadone, propoxyphene, and pentazocine, among others). "Houde is of the opinion that *morphine* is still the most satisfactory drug," Bonica had noted in 1953, and this view had not changed. Both Houde and Twycross agreed that opiate dosage should be titrated to patient pain, not to some predetermined standard. Both saw tolerance and physical dependence as manageable phenomena (although they disagreed on the probability of occurrence and methods of management). They agreed that adequate pain relief was achievable in almost all patients; but that proper management of pain and of the side effects of opiate use required close monitoring and physician involvement. As Twycross said, "REVIEW. REVIEW. REVIEW. REVIEW. REVIEW" (Twycross 1979a).

The work of both clinical research groups was reflected in the landmark WHO guidelines, published as *Cancer Pain Relief*, which described the use of strong opiates as a responsible and well-validated method of pain management. This booklet challenged accepted medical practices and legal controls on opiate use in countries around the world, including the United States; Jan Stjernswärd has recalled that the head of the WHO Publications Unit was so concerned at its recommendations that he delayed its release for 2 years (Joranson 1993; Tansey, in press). Moreover, the booklet challenged the imagined narrative that associated morphine with irrational euphoria, with a loss of control, with the end of life (although the guidelines addressed the management of the dying patient). The patient described in *Cancer Pain Relief* receives a systematic and methodically progressive course of analgesic treatment, epitomized by the metaphor of the ladder. The physician trusts the patient's report of pain as rational and reliable and prescribes "strong opioids" on the basis of clearly defined criteria. He or she assists the patient to maintain selfhood and quality of life by ongoing review and management of pain, side effects, and well-being (World Health Organization 1986).

The reimagined narrative of opiate practice as rational and affirmative developed in two very different research programs; in both settings, the social context of practice validated the patient as well as the research. It is easy to see this validation at work at St. Christopher's. The goal of pain management was to give the patient "new hope and incentive." so that he or she could "begin to live again … Freed from the day- and nightmare of constant pain, his last weeks or months take on a new look" (Twycross 1979b). It was the patient who suffered from the "day- and nightmare of constant pain" who could not control his or her life, who had lost his or her mental and emotional equilibrium. Cicely Saunders and her hospice staff used opiates to restore the patient's life and humanity. Research on the most appropriate drugs and methods started from this premise.

Houde and Rogers' work was focused on the comparison of analgesics; their starting premise was that the superior drug would be the one with the least narcotic effect, that still relieved pain effectively. But their methods, using each patient as "his own control," depended heavily on the accuracy of the patient's report of pain intensity, duration of relief, and occurrence of side effects. The active participation of the research subjects—"this group of heroic patients," as Richard Payne and Kathleen Foley (1984) have described them—and their ability to discriminate between drugs and to make rational statements were essential to the accuracy of the study results. The researchers' close involvement with many thousands of such patients enabled them to differentiate euphoria from well-being and to see each individual as a whole person, neither enslaved nor demoralized by opiates, but in need of understanding and relief from suffering.

EVIDENCE AND PRACTICE CHANGE

What of that other narrative—addiction, the "hideous spectacle"? Twycross's evidence that dependence was manageable among the terminally ill was impressive, but textbook writers had for many years endorsed opiate use in this specific population—in patients understood to be in their last days of life. There were other attempts to separate the story of the pain patient receiving opiates over the long term from that of the irrational abuser and addict. Many writers cited the finding of Jane Porter and Herschel Jick (1980) that only 0.03% of 11,882 patients (four individuals) given narcotics for pain at Boston University Hospital developed signs of addiction. This observation, however, briefly reported in a one-paragraph letter to the *New England Journal of Medicine*, was rather a fragile foundation for substantial practice change.

Richard Kanner and Kathleen Foley (1981) undertook a retrospective study of the 103 patients who came to the Sloan-Kettering Pain Clinic in a 2-year period (1977–1978). Among the 45 cancer patients still receiving opiates after 6 months, they found "no evidence of abuse"; "escalation of their drug intake," when it occurred, "was associated with rapidly progressive disease." Further, only 2 of the 17 noncancer patients receiving narcotics escalated their dosage and took more than the amount prescribed; both of these individuals were participants in the alternate narrative, presenting with "a long history of drug abuse behavior" (Kanner and Foley 1981). After further observations, Foley wrote emphatically:

> There are *no published long-term data* to support the thesis that chronic use of narcotic analgesics causes addiction. … Analysis of the patterns of drug intake in our series of cancer patients suggests that drug abuse and drug addiction should not be the primary concern of the prescribing physician. Our data suggest that drug use alone is not the major factor in the development of addiction, but other medical, social, and economic conditions seem to play an important role. (Foley 1981)

Foley's clinical reports paralleled contemporary analyses from the field of addiction studies, where physicians and psychiatrists were revising the etiological model. Since the work of Lawrence Kolb in the 1920s, the American addict had generally been considered a person with a severe personality defect and with little hope of cure, unable to control his or her craving for the drug-induced sensations of euphoria that relieved or masked psychological inadequacy (Kolb 1925). There were few challenges to this model or narrative while most habitual drug users were assumed to be members of racial minorities or of the lower socioeconomic classes. When drug abuse became more common among white, middle-class youth, Vietnam veterans, and urban professionals in the 1960s and 1970s, intense public and government concern encouraged and supported new research. The new model emerging in the 1980s emphasized a multifactorial etiology—genetic, psychological, and social—interacting with a pattern of learned behavior leading to compulsive drug use. Addiction specialists now put less emphasis on the drug's effects or the user's defects than on the behavior pattern; behavior that had been learned could be modified, adjusted, and perhaps unlearned (Acker 1993). The implied narrative readily correlated with one of expert clinical management of drug use in the pain patient.

Russell Portenoy and Kathleen Foley tried another retrospective review in the 1980s, this one of 38 noncancer patients who had received opiate analgesics for pain. They again found only two patients in the series, both with prior histories of abuse, who showed evidence of dependence or excessive use (Portenoy and Foley 1986). On the one hand, this study provided more positive evidence for a narrative of the pain patient who can learn to be a safe and sane user of opiates. On the other, there is the suggestion that the former drug abuser is still excluded or written out of the story.

Only 24 of the patients in this review, however, reported acceptable pain relief, and Portenoy and Foley could not identify any psychological or social variables in the patients that correlated highly with the success of treatment. But they found that a significant factor, perhaps the most significant, was "the intensive involvement of a single physician" responsible for the patient's overall care. This observation, in a different population and context, echoes the evidence from the Houde/Rogers and Twycross studies, that physician involvement with and acceptance of the patient is central to the effective rewriting of the imagined narrative of opiate use.

Twenty years after the WHO analgesic ladder was developed, the methodology has become known around the world and accepted in principle as a standard for the management of pain in cancer patients; but, as the work of Jan Stjernswärd and David Joranson (1995) and of June Dahl (this volume) illustrates, change in clinical practice has been slower to achieve. If opiate use is considered as a practice enmeshed in cultural narrative, as suggested here, the dilatory pace may be easier to understand. The most effective strategy for change, apparently, has been personal conversion; examples are Cicely Saunders' presentations of patient stories to medical student audiences (Faull and Nicholson, this volume) and the Role Model program developed by the American Alliance of Cancer Pain Initiatives (Dahl, this volume). Teaching the new model to a colleague, sharing experiences with individual patients on opiates, may be a more effective method of transmission for *a cultural narrative* than a didactic or prescriptive text.

THE NEW PATIENTS AND THEIR STORIES

The new narrative of opioid use is complicated, moreover, by the introduction of new protagonists—not only the patient with the history of drug use, but the cancer patient who will live longer and face multiple fluctuations in the course of the disease, as well as new and more stressful therapies. Their stories will be different from the stories of those told on the wards of James Ewing Hospital, or at St. Christopher's Hospice.

New kinds of narratives for these patients are evolving out of new experiences and new research. A recent example is the project of Steven Passik and colleagues (2000) to describe the willingness of 52 cancer patients and 111 women with HIV/AIDS to endorse aberrant drug-taking behaviors, in an effort to develop useful assessment tools for the physician managing pain in the current or former drug user. Another is Nessa Coyle's work in eliciting and analyzing cancer patients' stories of their experiences (this volume). These patient narratives reflect the persistence of the images of loss of control and loss of humanity associated with the use of opiates to relieve pain. A majority of the cancer patients in Passik's study, for example, thought that 25–50% of their peers got "high" or euphoric from their medication; many of the women with HIV/AIDS believed this to be the case with 50–75%. "[M]any patients believe that using illicit drugs for pain control ... and getting 'high' from pain medications are common behaviors. ... Patients do not seem to generalize from their own behavior to that of pain patients in general" (Passik et al. 2000).

Coyle's subjects associated opiate use with sleepiness or mental confusion, although they also perceived it as a blessing as death approached. As one said, "on the one hand, I have less pain with more medicine, but on the other hand, I'm not quite there, and I guess I prefer to be quite there, you know, because the sleeping is horrible ... basically it's like giving up" (Coyle, this volume). These last studies suggest that many patients have internalized the traditional narrative and the perceived value of maintaining control and resisting strong opiates (although others may not), at least until their last days. If physicians are to manage chronic or recurrent pain with opiates with the greatest efficacy and the least risk, they must not only imagine a new narrative for their patients, but also listen to the patients' internal narratives and teach them the new story to help them achieve well-being without losing their sense of selfhood to the property of euphoria.

REFERENCES

Acker CJ. Stigma or legitimation? A historical examination of the social potentials of addiction disease models. *J Psychoactive Drugs* 1993; 25:193–205.

Bonica JJ. *The Management of Pain*. Philadelphia: Lea and Febiger, 1953.

Bouchard R, Owens NF. *Nursing Care of the Cancer Patient*. St. Louis: Mosby, 1972.

Cole WH. Foreword. In: Schiffrin MJ (Ed). *The Management of Pain in Cancer*. Chicago: Year Book, 1956, pp 7–8.

Foley KM. Current issues in the management of cancer pain: Memorial Sloan-Kettering Cancer Center. *NIDA Res Monogr* May 1981; 36:169–181.

German CPH. *The Cancer Unit: An Ethnography*. Wakefield, MA: Nursing Resources, 1979.

Houde RW. Systemic analgesics and related drugs: narcotic analgesics. In: Bonica JJ, Ventafridda V (Eds). *International Symposium on Pain of Advanced Cancer*, Advances in Pain Research and Therapy, Vol. 2. New York: Raven Press, 1979, pp 263–273, 302.

Houde RW. Oral History Interview, conducted by Meldrum ML. Los Angeles: John C. Liebeskind History of Pain Collection, UCLA, 1995.

Hunt JM, Stollar TD, Littlejohns DW, Twycross RG, Vere DW. Patients with protracted pain: a survey conducted at the London Hospital. *J Med Ethics* 1977; 3:61–73.

Jacox AK. *Pain: A Source Book for Nurses and Other Health Professionals*. Boston: Little, Brown, 1977.

Joranson DE. Availability of opioids for cancer pain: recent trends, assessment of system barriers, new World Health Organization guidelines, and the risk of diversion. *J Pain Symptom Manage* 1993; 8:353–360.

Kanner RM, Foley KM. Patterns of narcotic drug use in a cancer pain clinic. *Ann New York Acad Sci* 1981; 362:161–172.

Kolb L. Types and characteristics of drug addicts. *Mental Hygiene* 1925; 9:300–313.

Marks RM, Sachar EJ. Undertreatment of medical inpatients with narcotic analgesics. *Ann Intern Med* 1973; 78:173–181.

Modell W, Houde RW. Factors influencing the clinical evaluation of drugs, with special reference to the double-blind technique. *JAMA* 1958; 167:2190–2199.

Nealon TF JR. *Management of the Patient with Cancer*. Philadelphia: W.B. Saunders, 1965.

Passik SD, Kirsh KL, McDonald MV, et al. A pilot survey of aberrant drug-taking attitudes and behaviors in samples of cancer and AIDS patients. *J Pain Symptom Manage* 2000; 19:274–286.

Payne R, Foley KM. Advances in the management of cancer pain. *Cancer Treatment Reports* 1984; 68:173–183.

Portenoy RK, Foley KM. Chronic use of opioid analgesia in non-malignant pain: report of 38 cases. *Pain* 1986; 25:171–186.

Porter J, Jick H. Addiction rare in patients treated with narcotics. *N Engl J Med* 1980; 302:123.

Reeves RB. A study of terminal patients. *J Pastoral Care* 1960; 14:218–223.

Rogers AG. Sociological and nursing aspects of cancer pain. In: Bonica JJ, Ventafridda V (Eds). *International Symposium on Pain of Advanced Cancer*, Advances in Pain Research and Therapy, Vol. 2. New York: Raven Press, 1979, pp 103–112.

Rogers AG. Oral History Interview, conducted by Meldrum ML. Los Angeles: John C. Liebeskind History of Pain Collection, 1995.

Saunders C. Oral History Interview, conducted by Liebeskind JC. Los Angeles: John C. Liebeskind History of Pain Collection, 1993.

Schiffrin MJ, Gross EG. Systemic analgesics. In: Schiffrin MJ (Ed). *The Management of Pain in Cancer.* Chicago: Year Book, 1956, pp 13–33.

Stjernswärd J, Joranson DE. Opioid availability and cancer pain: an unnecessary tragedy. *Support Care Cancer* 1995; 3:157–158.

Tansey EM. *Wellcome Witness Seminar on Pain Management.* London: Wellcome Institute, in press.

Twycross RG. Choice of strong analgesic in terminal cancer: Diamorphine or morphine? *Pain* 1977; 3:93–104.

Twycross RG. The Brompton Cocktail. In: Bonica JJ, Ventafridda V (Eds). *International Symposium on Pain of Advanced Cancer,* Advances in Pain Research and Therapy, Vol. 2. New York: Raven Press, 1979a, pp 291–300.

Twycross RG. Overview of analgesia. In: Bonica JJ, Ventafridda V (Eds). *International Symposium on Pain of Advanced Cancer,* Advances in Pain Research and Therapy, Vol. 2. New York: Raven Press, 1979b, pp 617–633.

World Health Organization. WHO Expert Committee on Drugs Liable to Produce Addiction. *Report on the 2nd Session, Geneva, January 9–14, 1950.* WHO Technical Report Series 21, 1950.

World Health Organization. *Cancer Pain Relief.* Geneva: World Health Organization, 1986.

Correspondence to: Marcia L. Meldrum, PhD, Department of History, Bunche 6265, Box 951473, University of California, Los Angeles, Los Angeles, CA 90095-1473, USA. Email: meldrum@history.ucla.edu.

Index

Progress in Pain Research and Management Series